Left Atrial Appendage

Editors

DHANUNJAYA LAKKIREDDY
DAVID R. HOLMES Jr
SAIBAL KAR

CARDIAC ELECTROPHYSIOLOGY CLINICS

www.cardiacEP.theclinics.com

Consulting Editors
RANJAN K. THAKUR
ANDREA NATALE

March 2020 • Volume 12 • Number 1

ELSEVIER

1600 John F. Kennedy Boulevard • Suite 1800 • Philadelphia, Pennsylvania, 19103-2899

http://www.theclinics.com

CARDIAC ELECTROPHYSIOLOGY CLINICS Volume 12, Number 1
March 2020 ISSN 1877-9182, ISBN-13: 978-0-323-75843-7

Editor: Stacy Eastman
Developmental Editor: Donald Mumford

Cardiac Electrophysiology Clinics (ISSN 1877-9182) is published quarterly by Elsevier Inc., 360 Park Avenue South, New York, NY 10010-1710. Months of issue are March, June, September, and December. Subscription prices are $231.00 per year for US individuals, $388.00 per year for US institutions, $249.00 per year for Canadian individuals, $438.00 per year for Canadian institutions, $303.00 per year for international individuals, $469.00 per year for international institutions and $100.00 per year for US, Canadian and international students/residents. To receive student/resident rate, orders must be accompanied by name of affilliated institution, date of term, and the signature of program/residency coordinator on institution letterhead. Orders will be billed at individual rate until proof of status is received. Foreign air speed delivery is included in all Clinics subscription prices. All prices are subject to change without notice. **POSTMASTER:** Send address changes to Cardiac Electrophysiology Clinics, Elsevier Health Sciences Division, Subscription Customer Service, 3251 Riverport Lane, Maryland Heights, MO 63043. **Customer Service: 1-800-654-2452 (US and Canada). From outside of the US and Canada, call 314-477-8871. Fax: 314-447-8029. E-mail: JournalsCustomerService-usa@elsevier.com (for print support); JournalsOnlineSupport-usa@elsevier.com (for online support).**

Reprints. For copies of 100 or more of articles in this publication, please contact the Commercial Reprints Department, Elsevier Inc., 360 Park Avenue South, New York, NY 10010-1710. Tel.: 212-633-3874; Fax: 212-633-3820; E-mail: reprints@elsevier.com.

Cardiac Electrophysiology Clinics is covered in *MEDLINE/PubMed (Index Medicus).*

Contributors

CONSULTING EDITORS

RANJAN K. THAKUR, MD, MPH, MBA, FHRS
Professor of Medicine and Director, Arrhythmia
Service, Thoracic and Cardiovascular Institute,
Sparrow Health System, Michigan State
University, Lansing, Michigan, USA

ANDREA NATALE, MD, FACC, FHRS
Executive Medical Director, Texas Cardiac
Arrhythmia Institute, St. David's Medical
Center, Austin, Texas; Consulting Professor,
Division of Cardiology, Stanford University,
Palo Alto, California; Adjunct Professor of
Medicine, Heart and Vascular Center, Case
Western Reserve University, Cleveland, Ohio;
Director, Interventional Electrophysiology,
Scripps Clinic, San Diego, California; Senior
Clinical Director, EP Services, California Pacific
Medical Center, San Francisco, California, USA

EDITORS

**DHANUNJAYA LAKKIREDDY, MD, FACC,
FHRS**
Executive Medical Director, Kansas City Heart
Rhythm Institution and Research Foundation,
Professor of Medicine, University of Missouri-
Columbia HCA MIDWEST HEALTH, Overland
Park, Kansas, USA

DAVID R. HOLMES Jr, MD, MACC
Consultant, Department of Cardiovascular
Diseases, Mayo Clinic, Rochester, Minnesota,
USA

SAIBAL KAR, MD
Professor of Medicine at David Geffen School
of Medicine at UCLA, Los Angeles, California,
USA; Director of Structural Heart Disease
Interventions & Research, Los Robles Regional
Medical Center, Thousand Oaks, Bakersfield
Heart Hospital, Bakersfield, California, USA

AUTHORS

ASHKAN AHMADIAN-TEHRANI, MD
Department of Medicine, Division of
Internal Medicine, The University of Texas
Health Science Center, San Antonio,
Texas, USA

KRISHNA AKELLA, DO
Arrhythmia Research Fellow, Kansas City
Heart Rhythm Institute (KCHRI) @ HCA
MidWest, Overland Park Regional Medical
Center, Overland Park, Kansas, USA

AMIN AL-AHMAD, MD
Texas Cardiac Arrhythmia Institute, St. David's
Medical Center, Austin, Texas, USA

MOHAMAD ALKHOULI, MD
Department of Cardiovascular Diseases, Mayo
Clinic, Rochester, Minnesota, USA

ANISH AMIN, MD
OhioHealth Riverside Methodist Hospital,
Columbus, Ohio, USA

ALISARA ANANNAB, MD
Texas Cardiac Arrhythmia Institute, St. David's
Medical Center, Austin, Texas, USA;
Department of Cardiovascular Intervention,
Central Chest Institute of Thailand, Nonthaburi,
Thailand

ARASH ARSHI, MD
OhioHealth Riverside Methodist Hospital,
Columbus, Ohio, USA

MOHAMED BASSIOUNY, MD
Texas Cardiac Arrhythmia Institute, St. David's
Medical Center, Austin, Texas, USA

LUCAS V.A. BOERSMA, MD, PhD
Cardiologist (Electrophysiologist), Professor,
Department of Cardiology, St. Antonius
Hospital, Nieuwegein, The Netherlands

STEFANO BORDIGNON, MD
Cardioangiologisches Centrum Bethanien,
AGAPLESION Markus Krankenhaus, Frankfurt/
Main, Germany

QIONG CHEN, MD
Texas Cardiac Arrhythmia Institute, St. David's
Medical Center, Austin, Texas, USA

SHAOJIE CHEN, MD
Cardioangiologisches Centrum Bethanien,
AGAPLESION Markus Krankenhaus, Frankfurt/
Main, Germany

DONATELLO CIRONE, MPH
Azienda Ospedaliero-Universitaria Careggi,
Florence, Italy

OLE DE BACKER, MD, PhD
Department of Cardiology, Heart Center,
Rigshospitalet, University of Copenhagen,
Copenhagen, Denmark

DOMENICO G. DELLA ROCCA, MD
Fellow, Texas Heart Rhythm Institute,
Department of Biomedical Engineering,
University of Texas, Texas Cardiac Arrhythmia
Institute, St. David's Medical Center, Austin,
Texas, USA

LUIGI DI BIASE, MD, PhD
Texas Cardiac Arrhythmia Institute, St. David's
Medical Center, Department of Internal
Medicine, Dell Medical School, University of
Texas, Department of Biomedical Engineering,
Cockrell School of Engineering, University of
Texas, Austin, Texas, USA; Arrhythmia
Services, Department of Medicine, Montefiore
Medical Center, Albert Einstein College of
Medicine, Bronx, New York, USA; Department
of Clinical and Experimental Medicine,
University of Foggia, Foggia, Italy

**JAMES R. EDGERTON, MD, FACS, FACC,
FHRS**
Senior Clinical Scientist, Department of
Epidemiology, Baylor Scott and White Health,
Dallas, Texas, USA

CHRISTOPHER R. ELLIS, MD, FACC, FHRS
Associate Professor of Medicine, Director, LAA
Closure Program, Vanderbilt Heart and
Vascular Institute, Vanderbilt University
Medical Center, Nashville, Tennessee, USA

MOTOKI FUKUTOMI, MD
Department of Cardiology, Heart Center,
Rigshospitalet, University of Copenhagen,
Copenhagen, Denmark

CAROLA GIANNI, MD, PhD
Texas Cardiac Arrhythmia Institute, St. David's
Medical Center, Austin, Texas, USA

THOMAS S. GILHOFER, MD
Interventional Cardiology, Division of
Cardiology, Vancouver General Hospital,
University of British Columbia, Vancouver,
British Columbia, Canada

**RAKESH GOPINATHANNAIR, MD, FACC,
FHRS**
Cardiac Electrophysiology Laboratory Director,
Kansas City Heart Rhythm Institute (KCHRI) @
HCA MidWest, Regional Medical Center,
Overland Park, Kansas, USA

DAVID R. HOLMES Jr, MD, MACC
Consultant, Department of Cardiovascular
Diseases, Mayo Clinic, Rochester, Minnesota,
USA

RODNEY P. HORTON, MD
Texas Cardiac Arrhythmia Institute, St. David's
Medical Center, Austin, Texas, USA

GREGORY G. JACKSON, MD
Internal Medicine Residency Program,
Vanderbilt University Medical Center,
Nashville, Tennessee, USA

SAMIR R. KAPADIA, MD
Chairman, Department of Cardiovascular Medicine, Cleveland Clinic, Cleveland, Ohio, USA

AMAR KRISHNASWAMY, MD
Program Director, Interventional Cardiology, Cleveland Clinic, Cleveland, Ohio, USA

DHANUNJAYA LAKKIREDDY, MD, FACC, FHRS
Executive Medical Director, Kansas City Heart Rhythm Institution and Research Foundation, Professor of Medicine, University of Missouri-Columbia HCA MIDWEST HEALTH, Overland Park, Kansas, USA

RANDALL J. LEE, MD, PhD
Department of Electrophysiology, University of California, San Francisco, San Francisco, California, USA

MONIEK MAARSE, MD
PhD Candidate, Department of Cardiology, St. Antonius Hospital, Department E1 R&D Cardiology, St. Antonius Hospital, Nieuwegein, The Netherlands

BRYAN MACDONALD, MD
Texas Cardiac Arrhythmia Institute, St. David's Medical Center, Austin, Texas, USA

SANGHAMITRA MOHANTY, MD
Texas Cardiac Arrhythmia Institute, St. David's Medical Center, Austin, Texas, USA

GHULAM MURTAZA, MD
Arrhythmia Research Fellow, Kansas City Heart Rhythm Institute (KCHRI) @ HCA MidWest, Overland Park Regional Medical Center, Overland Park, Kansas, USA

ANDREA NATALE, MD, FACC, FHRS
Executive Medical Director, Texas Cardiac Arrhythmia Institute, St. David's Medical Center, Austin, Texas; Consulting Professor, Division of Cardiology, Stanford University, Palo Alto, California; Adjunct Professor of Medicine, Heart and Vascular Center, Case Western Reserve University, Cleveland, Ohio; Director, Interventional Electrophysiology, Scripps Clinic, San Diego, California; Senior Clinical Director, EP Services, California Pacific Medical Center, San Francisco, California, USA

ABDI RASEKH, MD
Associate Professor, Cardiology, Baylor College of Medicine, Associate Professor, Cardiology, Texas Heart Institute, Houston, Texas, USA

JORGE ROMERO, MD
Arrhythmia Services, Department of Medicine, Montefiore Medical Center, Albert Einstein College of Medicine, Bronx, New York, USA

KYOUNG RYUL JULIAN CHUN, MD
Cardioangiologisches Centrum Bethanien, AGAPLESION Markus Krankenhaus, Frankfurt/Main, Germany

PAYAM SAFAVI-NAEINI, MD
Research Associate, Electrophysiology Clinical Research and Innovation, Texas Heart Institute, Houston, Texas, USA

ANU SAHORE, MD
Texas Cardiac Arrhythmia Institute, St. David's Medical Center, Austin, Texas USA

CARLOS E. SANCHEZ, MD
OhioHealth Riverside Methodist Hospital, Columbus, Ohio, USA

JACQUELINE SAW, MD, FRCPC, FACC, FAHA, FSCAI, FSCCT
Interventional Cardiology, Division of Cardiology, Vancouver General Hospital, Clinical Professor, University of British Columbia, Vancouver, British Columbia, Canada

BORIS SCHMIDT, MD, FHRS
Cardioangiologisches Centrum Bethanien, AGAPLESION Markus Krankenhaus, Frankfurt/Main, Germany

LARS SØNDERGAARD, MD, DMSc
Department of Cardiology, Heart Center, Rigshospitalet, University of Copenhagen, Copenhagen, Denmark

MARTIN J. SWAANS, MD, PhD
Cardiologist (Imaging), Department of Cardiology, St. Antonius Hospital, Nieuwegein, The Netherlands

NICOLA TARANTINO, MD
Arrhythmia Services, Department of Medicine,
Montefiore Medical Center, Albert Einstein
College of Medicine, Bronx, New York, USA

CHINTAN TRIVEDI, MD, MPH
Texas Cardiac Arrhythmia Institute, St. David's
Medical Center, Austin, Texas, USA

ALEKSANDR VOSKOBOINIK, MBBS, PhD
Department of Electrophysiology, University of
California, San Francisco, San Francisco,
California, USA

OUSSAMA WAZNI, MD
Section Head, Cardiac Electrophysiology,
Cleveland Clinic, Cleveland, Ohio, USA

BEN WILKINS, MBChB
Department of Cardiology, Heart Center,
Rigshospitalet, University of Copenhagen,
Copenhagen, Denmark

STEVEN J. YAKUBOV, MD
Director, Advanced Structural Heart Disease,
Riverside Methodist Hospital, Columbus, Ohio,
USA

BHARATH YARLAGADDA, MD
Fellow, Department of Cardiology,
University of New Mexico, Albuquerque,
New Mexico,
USA

Contents

Atrial fibrillation (AF) has been a source of fascination for more than 100 years. Most early investigations centered on the mechanisms of the arrhythmia (reentry versus automaticity; site of origin; approaches to treatment or prevention; and the clinical consequences), specifically tachycardia-induced cardiomyopathy and the potential for lethal events in special circumstances (eg, preexcitation syndromes). The current increased interest in AF has been heightened by increasing information on the clinical volume and number of patients affected. Recent data identify a current prevalence rate of 6 million patients in the United States, which is predicted to become 12 million by 2030.

Atrial fibrillation (AF) is the most common arrhythmia. Patients with AF have a higher risk for thromboembolism than individuals without AF. The left atrial appendage (LAA) is the main source of thromboembolism because of its anatomic, mechanical, and electrophysiologic properties, and accounts for more than 90% of thrombus formation in patients with AF. Advancement in imaging expands knowledge about anatomic and physiologic characteristics of LAA. The risk of thromboembolism events in patients with AF depends on clinical comorbidities and structural and physiologic parameters of atria, especially LAA. This article discusses AF-related thromboembolic events and the role of the LAA.

The left atrial appendage (LAA) affects body homeostasis via atrial natriuretic peptide and the renin-angiotensin-aldosterone system and plays an important role in atrial compliance. Approximately 90% of clots in nonvalvular atrial fibrillation (AF) are formed in the LAA. AF is the most common sustained cardiac arrhythmia and is frequently associated with stroke. Because anticoagulation for stroke prophylaxis carries a higher bleeding risk, LAA closure via epicardial and endocardial approaches has gained popularity and is being increasingly pursued for arrhythmogenic, homeostatic, and stroke-reduction benefits. This review discusses the

computer tomography angiography, transesophageal echocardiography, or intra-cardiac echocardiography in conjunction with fluoroscopy has improved the efficacy, procedural success, and safety of left atrial appendage closure in recent years. Proceduralists need to familiarize themselves with the various modalities and understand their complimentary roles and their limitations.

Left atrial appendage closure (LAAC) is noninferior to oral vitamin K antagonist therapy for the reduction of nonvalvular atrial fibrillation-related stroke risk. Currently, the procedure is most widely accepted in patients who cannot tolerate oral anticoagulants. This patient population is generally comorbid, making any reduction in procedural complications paramount. LAAC has important complications described in the periprocedural and postprocedural periods. The prevention and management of complications regarding vascular access, transseptal puncture, pericardial effusion, device embolization, stroke, air embolusperidevice leak, device-related thrombus and device erosion/ late pericardial effusion are discussed.

Excluding the left atrial appendage in patients with nonvalvular atrial fibrillation is a mechanical way to decrease stroke risk. During endothelialization, the closure device is exposed to circulating blood, which might activate the coagulation cascade. In excessive proportions, possibly resulting in the development of device-related thrombus, requiring a bridging period with optimal antithrombotic treatment. Initial protocol treatment is less suitable for patients with contraindications to anticoagulation. Less intensive antithrombotic regimens investigated suggest safety and efficacy, however further research is required. A tailored treatment, considering bleeding and thromboembolic risk based on patient/procedural characteristics in every patient, is probably the best approach.

Left atrial appendage (LAA) is the dominant source of systemic thromboembolic (TE) events in patients with nonvalvular atrial fibrillation (AF). In patients with significant bleeding risk, various LAA exclusion strategies have been developed as an alternative to pharmacologic TE prophylaxis. Nevertheless, in a relatively small percentage of patients, incomplete LAA closure can be documented, either at the time of procedure or during follow-up. This persistent patency can potentially jeopardize an effective stroke prophylaxis. Hereby, we report an update on the current clinical implications of LAA leaks and how to manage them.

Left atrial appendage occlusion is an evolving technology with demonstrable benefits of stroke prophylaxis in patients with atrial fibrillation unsuitable for anticoagulation. This has resulted in the development of a plethora of transcatheter devices to achieve epicardial exclusion and endocardial occlusion. In this review, the authors summarize the differences in technique, target patient population, outcomes, and complication profiles of endocardial and epicardial techniques.

Left atrial appendage exclusion is efficacious for stroke prophylaxis in patients with atrial fibrillation. Surgical excision provides reliable left atrial appendage exclusion, whereas surgical occlusion does not. Specifically, 2-layer internal suture ligation has a high failure rate. Left atrial appendage exclusion concomitant to another cardiac surgical procedure is indicated in patients with atrial fibrillation but not in patients without baseline atrial fibrillation. Studies currently underway will further define the role of concomitant surgical left atrial appendage exclusion, especially for the population without baseline atrial fibrillation but at high risk of developing postoperative atrial fibrillation.

Interventional cardiologists and electrophysiologists perform various procedures to improve the quality and longevity of life. The mitigation of stroke risk in patients with atrial fibrillation may be ignored when considering other more acute or urgent situations, such as severe coronary or valvular heart disease requiring treatment or symptomatic atrial fibrillation necessitating ablation. However, we must keep this long-term stroke risk in mind to optimize patients' overall outcomes. Percutaneous left atrial appendage occlusion is an important option in those who present with high stroke and bleeding risk. Ongoing studies will help provide objective data in this arena.

Recent design changes for left atrial appendage (LAA) closure devices have led to significant improvement by facilitating the procedural workflow (no need for pigtail catheter-guided LAA intubation), moving the workspace from distal LAA to the landing zone (closed distal end design), and improving device stability (different anchor design). The availability of different device types (plug vs disc-lobe design) offers an option to tailor a device type to a patient's anatomy; thereby, sealing results have improved substantially. The issue of device-related thrombus has not been resolved and deserves future research, with the goal of eliminating postprocedural antithrombotic medication without increasing risk for stroke.

CARDIAC ELECTROPHYSIOLOGY CLINICS

SERIES OF RELATED INTEREST

Cardiology Clinics
Available at: https://www.cardiology.theclinics.com/

THE CLINICS ARE AVAILABLE ONLINE!
Access your subscription at:
www.theclinics.com

Foreword
Left Atrial Appendage Occlusion

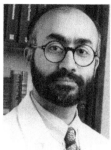
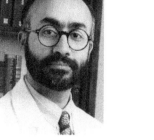

Ranjan K. Thakur, MD, MPH, MBA, FHRS   Andrea Natale, MD, FACC, FHRS
Consulting Editors

We are pleased to introduce this issue of *Cardiac Electrophysiology Clinics* focused on discussion of left atrial appendage occlusion for prevention of embolism in atrial fibrillation (AF).

The readership is well acquainted with the fact that cerebral embolism and other embolic events are some of the most dreaded complications of AF. Anticoagulation can significantly reduce this risk. However, some patients don't tolerate anticoagulation or are poor candidates for it. Stroke prevention can still be achieved in these patients by occluding or removing the left atrial appendage.

The appendage can be occluded surgically (at the time of a concomitant cardiac surgery) or via a number of devices. This issue of *Cardiac Electrophysiology Clinics* focuses on device-based prevention of embolism. Our knowledge continues to evolve as we learn more about the pathophysiology of AF, the physiologic/anatomic basis of thrombus formation, the association of AF with systemic vascular disease, the patient and appendage anatomic characteristics in whom the risk-benefit ratio is optimal for device-occlusion therapy, the role of the left atrial appendage in the pathogenesis of AF as well as its contribution to hemodynamics. An increasing number of devices have become available, and we have gained

follow-up data, so we now have information on device-related complications to help guide device selection and risk-benefit analysis.

This issue of *Cardiac Electrophysiology Clinics* has been edited by two interventional cardiologists and an electrophysiologist. We congratulate Drs Holmes, Kar, and Lakkireddy for bringing a balanced perspective to the readership. We hope the readership will find this issue useful and informative.

Ranjan K. Thakur, MD, MPH, MBA, FHRS
Sparrow Thoracic and Cardiovascular Institute
Michigan State University
1440 East Michigan Avenue, Suite 400
Lansing, MI 48912, USA

Andrea Natale, MD, FACC, FHRS
Texas Cardiac Arrhythmia Institute
Center for Atrial Fibrillation at
St. David's Medical Center
1015 East 32nd Street, Suite 516
Austin, TX 78705, USA

E-mail addresses:
thakur@msu.edu (R.K. Thakur)
andrea.natale@stdavids.com (A. Natale)

cardiacEP.theclinics.com

Preface

Left Atrial Appendage: What Do We Know? What Do We Need? Where Are We Going?

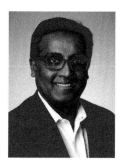   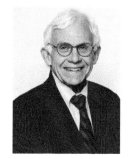   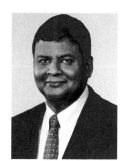

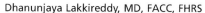

Dhanunjaya Lakkireddy, MD, FACC, FHRS   David R. Holmes Jr, MD, MACC   Saibal Kar, MD

Editors

Atrial fibrillation (AF) remains the focus of intense and increasing interest from multiple stakeholders, including family physicians, internists, general and interventional cardiologists, electrophysiologists, cardiovascular surgeons, and industry. This has been driven by the fact that it is the most common significant cardiac arrhythmia .with an estimated 6,000,000 patients by 2030. Its clinical consequences include, among others, the need for bradycardia support pacemakers as well as tachycardia-induced cardiomyopathy and stroke.

Within the past decade, there has been emphasis on pulmonary vein isolation for treatment and prevention of AF; more recently, another area of major interest has centered on stroke prevention. For the latter indication, the closely interrelated triad of increasing AF, increasing patient age, and increasing incidence of stroke has been documented repeatedly.

This issue focuses on the prevention of stroke for which an increasing amount of information has become available. New opportunities continue to develop as we learn more about the pathophysiology of AF itself, the physiologic/anatomic basis of thrombus formation, the association of AF with systemic vascular disease, the increasing number of devices for left atrial exclusion, the patient, and anatomic characteristics in whom the risk-benefit ratio is optimal, the role of the left atrial appendage in the pathogenesis of AF, and its role in hemodynamics. Finally, we now have information on the unanticipated effects of device exclusion with the documentation of device-related thrombus and its optimal treatment as well as screening.

This multidisciplinary field remains robust; the unmet clinical needs remain substantial, and the scientific rigor being devoted to understanding the fundamental issues and problem-solving promises continued great advances in the future.

Dhanunjaya Lakkireddy, MD, FACC, FHRS
The Kansas City Heart Rhythm Institution and
Research Foundation
HCA MIDWEST HEALTH
Second Floor, 5100 W 110th St
Overland Park, KS 66211, USA

David R. Holmes Jr, MD, MACC
Department of Cardiovascular Diseases
Mayo Clinic
200 First Street SouthWest
Rochester, MN 55905, USA

Saibal Kar, MD
David Geffen School of Medicine at UCLA
Structural Heart Disease Interventions & Research
Los Robles Regional Medical Center
227 W Janss Road, Suite 360
Thousand Oaks, CA 91360, USA

E-mail addresses:
dlakkireddy@gmail.com (D. Lakkireddy)
holmes.david@mayo.edu (D.R. Holmes)
saibalkar60@gmail.com (S. Kar)

Card Electrophysiol Clin 12 (2020) xv
https://doi.org/10.1016/j.ccep.2019.12.001
1877-9182/20/© 2019 Published by Elsevier Inc.

The History of the Left Atrial Appendage Occlusion

David R. Holmes Jr, MD, MACC*, Mohamad Alkhouli, MD

KEYWORDS

• Atrial fibrillation • Stroke prevention • Oral anticoagulation • Left atrial appendage occlusion

KEY POINTS

• In the setting of NVAF, the LAA has been found to be the source of thromboembolism in 90% of patients.
• Although the Watchman(tm) device is approved for use in both the US and European Union, there are differences in selection criteria. In contrast to the US, EU criteria does not require that the patient have a contraindication to anticoagulants.
• Device related thrombus in patients receiving a Watchman(tm) device occurs in approximately 4% of patients.

Atrial fibrillation (AF) has been a source of fascination for more than 100 years.[1] Most early investigations centered on the mechanisms of the arrhythmia (reentry versus automaticity; site of origin; approaches to treatment or, optimally, prevention; and, importantly, the clinical consequences), specifically tachycardia-induced cardiomyopathy and the potential for lethal events in special circumstances (eg, preexcitation syndromes). The current increased interest in AF has been heightened by the increasing information on the clinical volume and number of patients affected. Recent data identify a current prevalence rate of 6 million patients in the United States, which is predicted to increase to 12 million by 2030.[2,3]

Although past interest has focused on the pathophysiology of the arrhythmia, over the past several decades, the prominent association between AF and stroke/systemic embolization and its further association with advancing age has assumed a central role. In elderly patients, AF accounts for up to 20% to 40% of strokes, which tend to be larger and have an increased propensity for recurrence.[4–12] Given the magnitude of morbidity and mortality associated with stroke, which is now the third leading cause of death and the leading cause of disability in the United States, increased attention has been directed at risk prediction scores and prevention.

Early interest in the field was the result of surgical observations in patients undergoing treatment of rheumatic mitral valve disease because peripheral arterial emboli were common in that disease setting. Madden[13] in 1949 reported on 2 patients, a 32-year-old woman and a 52-year-old man in whom he "performed resection of the left auricular appendix...as prophylaxis for recurring arterial thrombi." In both patients, thrombi were found in that "auricular appendix". In the late 1940s and 1950s, in surgical series thrombi were identified in both the body of the left atrium as well as in the left auricular appendix (now known as the left atrial appendage [LAA]). Along with these findings came enhanced understanding of the complexity as well as the fragility of this structure, which has been termed "the most lethal human attachment because of its tendency to tear."[14] The relative role of the underlying disease state in the location of thrombus was evaluated and highlighted in an

Department of Cardiovascular Diseases, Mayo Clinic, 200 First Street Southwest, Rochester, MN 55905, USA
* Corresponding author.
E-mail address: Holmes.david@mayo.edu

Card Electrophysiol Clin 12 (2020) 1–11
https://doi.org/10.1016/j.ccep.2019.11.009
1877-9182/20/© 2019 Elsevier Inc. All rights reserved.

analysis of multiple published reports, including transesophageal echocardiography (TEE), autopsy, and operative reports by Blackshear and Odell.[15] These investigators found that, in patients with nonvalvular AF (NVAF), the origin of thrombi associated with stroke or systematic embolism was the LAA in 90% of cases; this contrasts in patients with valvular heart disease in whom thrombi were found in the body of the left atrium (LA) in approximately 60% of patients, with only approximately 40% found in the LAA. This seminal observation about differences in events and their association with specific pathophysiology has formed the basis for local site-specific therapy with LAA occlusion (LAAO), which has been carried forward to this day: namely that NVAF of the LAA is responsible for 90% of the pathophysiology of stroke/systemic embolization, whereas in valvular AF, specifically defined as mitral valve stenosis (either from rheumatic heart disease or mitral annular calcification, and/or mitral valve replacement with a mechanical valve), the thrombus is more commonly related to the body of the LA. A recent of study by Cresti and colleagues[16] corroborated this theory in a contemporary cohort by documenting that the location of LA thrombus was in the LAA in greater than 99% of AF patients who were found to have a thrombus on TEE.

With that as background, attention focused on LAAO for prevention of stroke/systemic embolization in those patients with NVAF at increased risk for those events. Given that not all patients with NVAF develop a stroke/systemic embolization, there has been development and widespread implementation of risk scores that can be used to guide therapy. Such risk scores are currently used as part of the risk prediction screening process, as well as recommendation for the procedure and requirement for its reimbursement. The most common is the CHA_2DS_2-VASc (congestive heart failure; hypertension; age ≥75 years; diabetes mellitus; prior stroke, transient ischemic attack, or thromboembolism; vascular disease; age 65–74 years; sex category) score,[17] which includes only clinical demographic characteristics and can identify a spectrum of patients in whom the predicted yearly incidence of stroke ranges from 1% to 20%. Although imperfect, such scores are now embedded in professional societal guidelines.

Based on surgical approaches to LAA occlusion or obliteration,[18,19] percutaneous strategies were developed. Throughout this time frame, the standards of care were anticoagulation: early on with vitamin K antagonists (VKAs) and subsequently with direct oral anticoagulants (DOACs).[5,20–26] Although effective, anticoagulation was often limited by clinical demographics, with patients having relative or absolute contraindications to anticoagulation. Although the specifics of defining relative versus absolute contraindications vary, they are both important in addressing the risk/benefit ratio. More recently, an equally large factor in developing and implementing strategies of care has been the increasing information related to the issue of noncompliance with long-term oral anticoagulation with VKAs but also with DOACs.[25,26] Accordingly, from the onset of site specific therapy, investigators have considered LAAO as an alternative to anticoagulant therapy for patients in whom anticoagulation was thought either to be not possible or not ideal for long-term treatment. A more optimal strategy that could be developed after accumulation of more scientifically controlled data is that patients with NVAF could be offered 2 potential strategic options: namely long-term anticoagulation or local site-specific therapy with a device.

The initial technology described was the percutaneous left atrial appendage transcatheter occluder (PLAATO), a self-expanding, balloon-shaped, nitinol cage that was covered on its left atrial surface with an occlusive polytetrafluoroethylene membrane. This device was placed via a percutaneous transseptal access into the LAA.[27,28] Stability was maintained by 3 rows of small anchors. Following in vivo canine animal models, human studies were initiated with the first implantation in 2001 followed by larger experiences in international as well as national multicenter studies. The 5-year results were reported by 2 working groups: North American and European registries.[27,28] In both of these registries, the observed stroke risk was less than the estimated annual risk rate obtained using risk prediction scores. This approach of comparing observed versus predicted rates of events has been used for all subsequent registries. With this strategy, in registries that do not include a control limb of patients, it allows evaluation of the efficacy of LAAO. After these promising results, because of economic issues related to regulatory hurdles and the cost of randomized clinical trials (RCTs), the PLAATO device was discontinued by the manufacturer.

During roughly the same time frame, a similar nitinol self-expanding cage covered on its atrial facing side with a biocompatible but semipermeable polymer surface membrane was developed. This device was also placed percutaneously after transseptal access in the LAA. Stability of this device was also enhanced with anchoring barbs. After satisfactory in vivo canine demonstration,[29] working closely with the US Food and Drug Administration (FDA), Atritech (the initial company involved in design, fabrication, and preclinical studies) initiated the first human clinical study in 2002 in Trier, Germany, followed by larger pilot studies in carefully selected patients.

After the pilot human experience and recognizing the clinical need, the next steps included the development of a randomized clinical trial in conjunction with the FDA. The company had never been involved in a clinical trial with this technology, although the staff had been well versed in the approaches required by virtue of their work with other device companies. Subsequently, the PROTECT AF (Watchman LAA System for Embolic Protection in Patients with Atrial Fibrillation) trial discussions were initiated involving industry, statisticians, regulatory agencies, and physicians.[30]

The need for randomization was central, but questions revolved around the focus of specific patient groups. The 2 options at that time were (1) patients in whom conventional therapy with anticoagulation (VKAs at that time) was contraindicated, or (2) patients who were acceptable candidates for chronic anticoagulation. The first possibility, although it was a large unmet clinical need, was difficult because identification of the control in the medical therapy limb was problematic in that there were no data on Plavix for prevention of stroke and because Aspirin (ASA) as monotherapy was not thought to an effective alternative in these patients at increased risk of stroke. As part of this, there was concern at that time that the control group regimen may not be acceptable to local institutional review boards. Accordingly, the trial focused on patients who could take VKAs. Other important considerations were statistical. Was this to have a primary end point of noninferiority, and, if so, what was a reasonable boundary? Given that there were no data on the Watchman as a new, unknown therapy, a noninferiority boundary for the primary composite end point was set at 2.0%. In retrospect, some clinicians have thought that this boundary was too wide. The specific elements of the composite used were of great importance, including stroke or systemic embolism and mortality.

These questions and discussion about specific end points for comparison continue to be relevant. The question raised was whether only ischemic strokes could or should be used as the primary end point because the Watchman device would only protect against strokes arising from thrombus in the LAA, or whether all strokes would be a better metric. Along this line, hemorrhagic strokes may typically occur with anticoagulant therapy; accordingly, some clinicians have thought that this should be the primary end point. In contrast, others have thought that all-cause total stroke rate would be the optimal primary end point.

Also, given that a composite would include mortality, was it sufficient to have all-cause mortality, or just cardiovascular mortality, and, if a stroke resulted in the mortality, would it be double counted as both a stroke and death? Other important issues addressed include periprocedural medical therapy. There had been limited animal data available,[29] but it suggested that it would take several weeks for endothelialization of the device to occur, and the recommendation in the absence of hard data was to continue VKAs for 6 weeks, at which time a TEE was performed to document outcome. This strategy of a 6-week outcome following implantation and the recommendation for 6 weeks of anticoagulant therapy and ASA was subsequently mandated in the instructions for use (IFU). Other questions were residual leak, how to define it, how to treat it, and what specific routine TEE follow-up schedule should be recommended. An important issue has been the extensive development and/or widespread use of DOACs in this setting rather than warfarin. However, at the time of the initial PROTECT AF trial design, DOACs were not in widespread clinical use and so the anticoagulation strategy by default was VKAs with conventional monitoring of International Normalized Ratio.

Following FDA panel evaluation of the results of PROTECT AF, despite a successful vote for approval (**Table 1**), the FDA recommended a second trial to obtain more data in higher-risk patients.[31,32] There was concern about early safety

Table 1 United States Food and Drug Administration circulatory panel voting			
	2009 Panel 4/23/09	2013 Panel 12/11/13	2014 Panel 10/8/14
For Approval	7–5	NA	NA
Safety	NA	13–1	12–0
Efficacy	NA	13–1	6–7 (chair voted to break tie)
Positive Benefit/ Risk Profile	NA	13–1	6–5 (1 abstain)

Abbreviation: NA, not available.
(*From* Waksman R, Pendyala LK. Overview of the Food and Drug Administration circulatory system devices panel meetings on WATCHMAN left atrial appendage closure therapy. *The American journal of cardiology.* 2015;115(3):378-384; with permission.)

issues, including cardiac tamponade and pericardial effusion, as well as procedural-related strokes. This second trial, PREVAIL (Prospective Randomized Evaluation of the Watchman LAA Closure Device in Patients with Atrial Fibrillation vs Long-term Warfarin Therapy), included 3 pre-specified end points and enrolled higher-risk patients. (The boundaries for noninferiority were changed from 2.0 seen with PROTECT AF to 1.75 for PREVAIL. This change had a significant implication. Had the same boundaries of 2.0 been used, PREVAIL would have been positive for the primary end point.) Unexpectedly, this second trial did not meet all 3 end points, the reasons for which were the source of significant conjecture and continuing debate. Once again, the votes were for positive safety and efficacy and a positive benefit/risk profile. Again, more data were requested by the FDA and these data documenting improved safety and longer-term efficacy then resulted in the third and final panel on October 8, 2014, and panel approval with subsequent full FDA approval in March 2015. In retrospect, the Watchman device is the only device that has required 3 FDA panels for the same indication submission in the history of the FDA, despite all 3 panels being positive. The process was lengthy, tortuous, labyrinthine, and expensive, with estimated incremental aggregate cost in excess of $200 million. During that time, multiple design issues were raised and addressed (**Box 1**). These issues are still relevant in the design and implementation of current LAA closure trials.

Following FDA approval, there was the necessary Centers for Medicare & Medicaid Services (CMS) evaluation with its requisite robust and lengthy comment period. This process resulted in a national coverage determination, February 8, 2016, and IFU (**Box 2**) and reimbursement requirements (**Box 3**). Of note, US and European indications for use vary (**Box 4**). In Europe, most patients considered for Watchman need to have contraindications to warfarin; accordingly, in the European experience, antiplatelet strategies with either single or dual antiplatelet agents predominate, in contrast with anticoagulation. As a result of these deliberations and processes, all patients were required to be enrolled in a national registry to continue to allow accrual of data once the device had been introduced into the broad clinical arena. In addition to the mandated national registry, patients had been enrolled in 2 companion continued access industry registries, which now have the longest data set of this technology out to 5 years. Since FDA approval and CMS reimbursement, patient enrollment in the United States has increased

---

Box 1
Design issues

- Patient population: anticoagulant contraindicated or not?
- Trial end points: all stroke versus ischemic stroke, composite or single
- Selection criteria
- Periprocedural medications
- Site selection
- Postprocedural testing
- Superiority versus noninferiority: frequentist versus bayesian

---

Box 2
March 2015 Watchman instructions for use

The Watchman device is indicated to reduce the risk of thromboembolism from the LAA in patients with nonvalvular AF who:

- Are at increased risk for stroke and systemic embolism based on $CHADS_2$ (congestive heart failure, hypertension, age, diabetes, prior stroke) or CHA_2DS_2-VASc scores and are recommended for anticoagulation therapy
- Are deemed by their physicians to be suitable for warfarin
- Have an appropriate rationale to seek a nonpharmacologic alternative to warfarin, taking into account the safety and effectiveness of the device compared with warfarin

---

Box 3
United States reimbursement status Centers for Medicare & Medicaid Services national coverage decision (February 8, 2016)

Criteria for coverage:

- CHADS2 score greater than or equal to 2 or CHA_2DS_2-VASc score greater than or equal to 3
- A formal shared decision-making interaction with an independent noninterventional physician using an evidence-based decision tool on oral anticoagulation in patients with NVAF
- Suitable for short-term warfarin but deemed unable to take long-term oral anticoagulation

<table>
<tr><td colspan="2">

Box 4

Watchman indications for use: comparison of United States and European Union

</td></tr>
<tr><td>

US Indication

</td><td>

European Union Indication

</td></tr>
<tr><td>

The Watchman device is indicated to reduce the risk of thromboembolism from the LAA in patients with nonvalvular AF who:

- Are at increased risk for stroke and systemic embolism based on $CHADS_2$ or CHA_2DS_2-VASc scores and are recommended for anticoagulation therapy

- Are deemed by their physicians to be suitable for warfarin; and

- Have an appropriate rationale to seek a nonpharmacologic alternative to warfarin, taking into account the safety and effectiveness of the device compared with warfarin

</td><td>

The Watchman LAA closure technology is intended to prevent thrombus embolization from the LAA and reduce the risk of life-threatening bleeding events in patients with nonvalvular AF who are eligible for anticoagulation therapy or who have a contraindication to anticoagulation therapy

</td></tr>
</table>

significantly using the IFU criteria. In 2019, it is anticipated that 30,000 procedures will be performed.

There is now a robust data set of these 2 RCTs, their accompanying registries out to 5 years, as well as large multinational registries on which to base conclusions[33–42] (**Fig. 1**).

1. Patient safety has continued to improve related to greater operator experience, modifications in the technology, and changes in implant technique. Specific changes included a softer tip guiding catheter and the mandated use of a pigtail when placing the guiding sheath, both of which decreased trauma to the wall of the LAA. The most recent aggregated data document that pericardial effusion/tamponade occurs in approximately 1.5% of patients, procedural-related stroke in 0.75%, and procedural mortality in less than 0.1% (**Fig. 2, Table 2**).

2. Procedural success rates have been stable at approximately 97% to 98%.

3. During follow-up:
   a. The Watchman procedure has similar efficacy overall to VKA in all strokes.
   b. Watchman implantation is associated with major reduction in hemorrhagic stroke, a significant reduction in bleeding, and an apparent significant improvement in survival.

There are still important issues to be addressed in the future, which include:

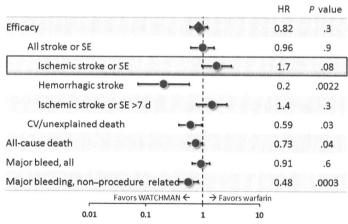

	HR	P value
Efficacy	0.82	.3
All stroke or SE	0.96	.9
Ischemic stroke or SE	1.7	.08
Hemorrhagic stroke	0.2	.0022
Ischemic stroke or SE >7 d	1.4	.3
CV/unexplained death	0.59	.03
All-cause death	0.73	.04
Major bleed, all	0.91	.6
Major bleeding, non–procedure related	0.48	.0003

Favors WATCHMAN ← | → Favors warfarin

0.01   0.1   1   10

Fig. 1. In a patient-level meta-analysis combining the randomized PROTECT AF and PREVAIL trial cohorts, patients receiving the Watchman device were compared with patients receiving chronic warfarin for major clinical end points. Hemorrhagic stroke was significantly reduced (hazard ratio [HR], 0.2), CV (cardiovascular) unexplained death reduced (HR, 0.59), and major nonprocedural related bleeding reduced (HR, 0.48). All-cause stroke in systemic embolism (SE) was similar for Watchman and control. (*From* Reddy VY, Doshi SK, Kar S, et al. 5-Year Outcomes After Left Atrial Appendage Closure: From the PREVAIL and PROTECT AF Trials. *Journal of the American College of Cardiology.* 2017;70(24):2964-2975; with permission.)

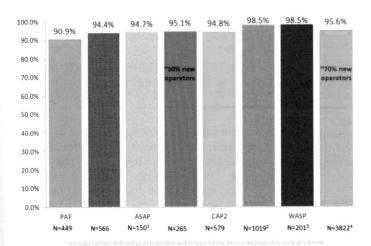

Fig. 2. Consistent procedural success. ASAP, ASA plavix feasibility study with WATCHMAN left atrial appendage closure technology; CAP2, continued access to PREVAIL registry; PAF, Paroxysmal Atrial Fibrillation; WASP, watchman in asian patients. (*Data from* Refs.[35,38,40,42])

a. Head-to-head comparison with novel oral anticoagulants.

b. Device-related thrombus (DRT), which occurs in approximately 4% of patients and seems to be associated with increased adverse events.[43–46] The optimal strategy for prevention of this, as well as treatment strategies once it has occurred, continues to evolve. As part of this, more information is needed about the pathophysiology. Several factors may play a role, including the metal connector pin, which is exposed to flowing blood and may serve as a nidus for thrombus formation or failure of the LA surface to completely endothelialize. In addition, the optimal surveillance strategy has not yet been identified. In some patients, the DRT appears within 3 months of the implant, whereas, in others, it does not appear until several months later. In this regard, the optimal detection strategy of thrombus continues to evolve with data now available for both TEE as well as computed tomography.

c. Ease of use. Given that the procedure will be performed by an increasing number of physicians, strategies for optimizing its safe and effective use are essential. The procedures have become safer, as documented (see **Fig. 2**, **Table 2**), but still carry the risk of all invasive approaches.

d. The need for early anticoagulation/dual antiplatelet therapy to facilitate device endothelialization. The use of early anticoagulation was identified in preclinical animal models, in which more complete endothelialization was not identified until approximately 1 to 2 months postimplant.[29] The need for this makes patient selection more problematic because some patients are at risk of bleeding

from anticoagulation even in the short term. Current RCTs are addressing this issue in patients randomized to Watchman versus a control group with ASA and Plavix. As previously mentioned, in Europe, the practice has changed to include either single or dual antiplatelet therapy postprocedure. Even with that approach, bleeding may occur in high-risk patients. New technology designed to address these issues with a nonthrombogenic coating, as well as the results of new RCTs that randomize patients unable to take even short-course anticoagulation versus only antiplatelet therapy, will continue to foster growth.

There are several other devices for LAAO (**Table 3**).[47–50] The one furthest along in terms of testing, development, implementation, and perhaps regulatory approval is the second-generation AMPLATZER device, Amulet. This device is based on iterative design changes from the earlier AMPLATZER Cardiac Plug device. The Amulet has a distal lobe that anchors the device in the landing zone in the LA, which is then attached to a proximal disc that seals the ostium. Similar to the Watchman device, it is placed after a transseptal procedure.

The Amulet has been the focus of a now-completed randomized head-to-head comparison with the Watchman device. The results of this trial will have important implications. There are also multiple outside of US registries focused on this device. The 1-year follow-up of the prospective global Amulet observational registry of 1088 patients has recently become available. Importantly in this registry study, 83% of patients had contraindications to anticoagulation.[47] Accordingly, in

Table 2
Comparison of procedural complications across Watchman studies

	PROTECT AF	PREVAIL	CAP	CAP2	EWOLUTION	After FDA Approval	Aggregate Data
Pericardial Tamponade	20 (4.3%)	5 (1.9%)	8 (1.4%)	11 (1.9%)	3 (0.29%)	39 (1.02%)	86 (1.28%)
Treated with Pericardiocentesis	13 (2.8%)	4 (1.5%)	7 (1.2%)	NA	2 (0.20%)	24 (0.63%)	—
Treated Surgically	7 (1.5%)	1 (0.4%)	1 (0.2%)	NA	1 (0.10%)	12 (0.31%)	—
Resulted in death	0	0	0	0	0	3 (0.78%)	—
Pericardial effusion: no intervention	4 (0.9%)	0	5 (0.9%)	3 (0.5%)	4 (0.39%)	11 (0.29%)	27 (0.40%)
Procedure-related Stroke	5 (1.15%)	1 (0.37%)	0	2 (0.35%)	1 (0.10%)	3 (0.078%)	12 (0.18%)
Device Embolization	3 (0.6%)	2 (0.7%)	1 (0.2%)	0	2 (0.20%)	9 (0.24%)	17 (0.25%)
Removed Percutaneously	1	0	0	0	1	3	—
Removed Surgically	2	2	1	0	1	6	—
Death							
Procedure-related Mortality	0	0	0	0	1 (0.1%)	3 (0.078%)	4 (0.06%)
Additional Mortality Within 7 days	0	0	0	1 (0.17%)	3 (0.29%)	1 (0.026%)	5 (0.07%)

Abbreviations: CAP, continued Access to PROTECT-AF; EWOLUTION, evaluating real-Life clinical outcomes in atrial fibrillation patients receiving the WATCHMAN left atrial appendage closure technology

Table 3
Endovascular left atrial appendage closure devices

Device Name	Company	Design	Device Sizes (mm)	Approval Status
Watchman	Boston Scientific	Single-lobe occlude with nitinol frame, PET membrane, 10 hooks	21, 24, 27, 30, 33	CE mark FDA approval
ACP	St Jude Medical	Lobe and disc (polyester mesh in both) nitinol mesh construct. Stabilizing wires	16, 18, 20, 22, 24, 26, 28, 30	CE mark
Amulet	St Jude Medical	Similar design to ACP, but wider lobe and disc, and more stabilizing wires	16, 18, 20, 22, 24, 26, 28, 30	CE mark
WaveCrest	Coherex Medical	Single-lobe occluder. Nitinol frame, polyurethane foam, ePTFE membrane, retractable anchors	22, 27, 32	CE mark
Occlutech LAA Occluder	Occlutech	Single-lobe occluder. Nitinol wire mesh, stabilizing loops, nanomaterial covering	15, 18, 21, 24, 27, 30, 33, 36, 39	CE mark
Sideris Transcatheter Patch	Custom Medical Devices	Frameless detachable latex balloon covered with polyurethane	—	NA
Lambre	Lifetech	Lobe and disc nitinol frame. PET membrane. Distal barb anchors	16–36	CE mark
pfm	pfm medical	Dual-disc nitinol frame (distal anchor, variable middle connector, proximal disc)	—	NA
Cardia	Cardia	Lobe and disc nitinol frame. Ivalon covering. Distal anchors	16, 20, 24, 28, 32	NA

Abbreviations: ACP, AMPLATZER cardiac plug; CE, Conformité Européene; ePTFE, expanded polytetrafluoroethylene; PET, polyethylene terephthalate.
Data from Hijazi ZMS, J. Nonpharmacologic therapy to prevent embolization in patients with atrial fibrillation. *UpTo Date.* 2019.;and Holmes DR Jr, Schwartz RS, Latus GC, Von Tassel RA. Intervent Cardiol Clin 7 (2018); 143-150.

contrast with the RCTs of Watchman, the patients were typically dismissed on only antiplatelet therapy (>80%).[47]

Procedural success was seen in 99% of cases during a mean follow-up of 11.1 ± 2.6 months. At 1 year, all-cause mortality was 8.4%, the observed ischemic stroke rate was 2.9%, and DRT was seen in 1.7%. Accordingly, the investigators concluded from this global perspective and registry of very high-risk stroke and bleeding patients that procedural success and 1-year follow-up is excellent despite the fact that only a minority of patients require anticoagulation.

The head-to-head RCT with Watchman will be important to identify similarities and differences between these two widely used devices. Multiple other endocardial devices are currently Conformité Européene (CE) mark approved or in

development and testing. All will follow the same path previously documented for Watchman and Amulet, with initial in vivo animal experiments, initial clinical experiences, and then RCTs. At the present time, at least in the United States, head-to-head trials will be required for FDA approval of any new LAAO devices.

The future for all of these devices will include common elements to be addressed:

1. Safety and early efficacy
   a. Minimizing procedural complications of pericardial effusion, device embolization, procedural bleeding, or stroke will be essential, as will high procedural or implant success rates
2. Long-term safety and efficacy
   a. Prevention or mitigation of stroke, both ischemic and hemorrhagic, realizing that

local site-specific therapy does not decrease ischemic strokes related to other vascular beds
  b. Prevention of DRT
  c. Minimizing device leak
  d. Documentation of need and efficacy of only single antiplatelet or dual antiplatelet therapy

Final and important issues will be:

1. Safety and efficacy of local site-specific therapy versus DOACs.
2. Comparative effectiveness of LAAO versus DOACs.
3. Resolution of DRT.
4. The need for anatomy-specific therapy. Anatomy-specific therapy has great implications given the large variety of anatomic shapes and sizes, and the three-dimensional origin and course of the LAA. There will be several devices to choose from; however, having all the potential devices available in the cardiac laboratory would be cost-prohibitive. Realistically, an approach might be to have 2 devices that together can cover the pool of patients with NVAF at increased risk for stroke.
5. The application of LAAO in concert with other structural heart procedures, such as transcatheter aortic valve replacement, MitraClip, and AF ablation.

CONFLICT OF INTEREST DISCLOSURES

None.

REFERENCES

1. Prystowsky EN. The history of atrial fibrillation: the last 100 years. J Cardiovasc Electrophysiol 2008; 19(6):575–82.
2. Kirchhof P, Benussi S, Kotecha D, et al. 2016 ESC guidelines for the management of atrial fibrillation developed in collaboration with EACTS. Rev Esp Cardiol (Engl Ed) 2017;70(1):50.
3. January CT, Wann LS, Calkins H, et al. 2019 AHA/ACC/HRS focused update of the 2014 AHA/ACC/HRS guideline for the management of patients with atrial fibrillation: a report of the American College of Cardiology/American Heart Association Task Force on clinical practice guidelines and the heart rhythm society. Heart Rhythm 2019;74(1):104–32.
4. Alkhouli M, Alqahtani F, Aljohani S, et al. Burden of atrial fibrillation-associated ischemic stroke in the United States. JACC Clin Electrophysiol 2018;4(5): 618–25.
5. Alkhouli M, Noseworthy PA, Rihal CS, et al. Stroke prevention in nonvalvular atrial fibrillation: a stakeholder perspective. J Am Coll Cardiol 2018;71(24): 2790–801.
6. Hayden DT, Hannon N, Callaly E, et al. Rates and determinants of 5-year outcomes after atrial fibrillation-related stroke: a population study. Stroke 2015;46(12):3488–93.
7. Heidbuchel H, Verhamme P, Alings M, et al. Updated European Heart Rhythm Association practical guide on the use of non-vitamin-K antagonist anticoagulants in patients with non-valvular atrial fibrillation: executive summary. Eur Heart J 2017;38(27): 2137–49.
8. Lip G, Freedman B, De Caterina R, et al. Stroke prevention in atrial fibrillation: past, present and future. Comparing the guidelines and practical decision-making. Thromb Haemost 2017;117(7):1230–9.
9. Lip GYH, Brechin CM, Lane DA. The global burden of atrial fibrillation and stroke: a systematic review of the epidemiology of atrial fibrillation in regions outside North America and Europe. Chest 2012; 142(6):1489–98.
10. Oldgren J, Healey JS, Ezekowitz M, et al. Variations in cause and management of atrial fibrillation in a prospective registry of 15,400 emergency department patients in 46 countries: the RE-LY Atrial Fibrillation Registry. Circulation 2014; 129(15):1568–76.
11. Schnabel RB, Yin X, Gona P, et al. 50 year trends in atrial fibrillation prevalence, incidence, risk factors, and mortality in the Framingham Heart Study: a cohort study. Lancet 2015;386(9989):154–62.
12. Wolf PA, Abbott RD, Kannel WB. Atrial fibrillation as an independent risk factor for stroke: the Framingham Study. Stroke 1991;22(8):983–8.
13. Madden JL. Resection of the left auricular appendix; a prophylaxis for recurrent arterial emboli. J Am Med Assoc 1949;140(9):769–72.
14. Johnson WD, Ganjoo AK, Stone CD, et al. The left atrial appendage: our most lethal human attachment! Surgical implications. Eur J Cardiothorac Surg 2000;17(6):718–22.
15. Blackshear JL, Odell JA. Appendage obliteration to reduce stroke in cardiac surgical patients with atrial fibrillation. Ann Thorac Surg 1996;61(2):755–9.
16. Cresti A, Garcia-Fernandez MA, Sievert H, et al. Prevalence of extra-appendage thrombosis in non-valvular atrial fibrillation and atrial flutter in patients undergoing cardioversion: a large transoesophageal echo study. EuroIntervention 2019;15(3): e225–30.
17. Friberg L, Rosenqvist M, Lip GY. Evaluation of risk stratification schemes for ischaemic stroke and bleeding in 182 678 patients with atrial fibrillation: the Swedish Atrial Fibrillation cohort study. Eur Heart J 2012;33(12):1500–10.

18. Cox JL. Mechanical closure of the left atrial appendage: is it time to be more aggressive? J Thorac Cardiovasc Surg 2013;146(5):1018–27.e2.

19. Emmert MY, Puippe G, Baumuller S, et al. Safe, effective and durable epicardial left atrial appendage clip occlusion in patients with atrial fibrillation undergoing cardiac surgery: first long-term results from a prospective device trial. Eur J Cardiothorac Surg 2014;45(1):126–31.

20. Holmes DR Jr, Alkhouli M, Reddy V. Left atrial appendage occlusion for the unmet clinical needs of stroke prevention in nonvalvular atrial fibrillation. Mayo Clin Proc 2019;94(5):864–74.

21. Holmes DR Jr, Reddy VY. Left atrial appendage and closure: who, when, and how. Circ Cardiovasc Interv 2016;9(5):e002942.

22. Hsu JC, Maddox TM, Kennedy KF, et al. Oral anticoagulant therapy prescription in patients with atrial fibrillation across the spectrum of stroke risk: insights from the NCDR PINNACLE registry. JAMA Cardiol 2016;1(1):55–62.

23. Ruff CT, Giugliano RP, Braunwald E, et al. Comparison of the efficacy and safety of new oral anticoagulants with warfarin in patients with atrial fibrillation: a meta-analysis of randomised trials. Lancet 2014; 383(9921):955–62.

24. Vinereanu D, Lopes RD, Bahit MC, et al. A multifaceted intervention to improve treatment with oral anticoagulants in atrial fibrillation (IMPACT-AF): an international, cluster-randomised trial. Lancet 2017;390(10104):1737–46.

25. Yao X, Abraham NS, Alexander GC, et al. Effect of Adherence to oral anticoagulants on risk of stroke and major bleeding among patients with atrial fibrillation. J Am Heart Assoc 2016;5(2).

26. Yao X, Shah ND, Sangaralingham LR, et al. Non-vitamin K antagonist oral anticoagulant dosing in patients with atrial fibrillation and renal dysfunction. J Am Coll Cardiol 2017;69(23):2779–90.

27. Ostermayer SH, Reisman M, Kramer PH, et al. Percutaneous left atrial appendage transcatheter occlusion (PLAATO system) to prevent stroke in high-risk patients with non-rheumatic atrial fibrillation: results from the international multi-center feasibility trials. J Am Coll Cardiol 2005;46(1):9–14.

28. Bayard YL, Omran H, Neuzil P, et al. PLAATO (Percutaneous Left Atrial Appendage Transcatheter Occlusion) for prevention of cardioembolic stroke in non-anticoagulation eligible atrial fibrillation patients: results from the European PLAATO study. EuroIntervention 2010;6(2):220–6.

29. Schwartz RS, Holmes DR, Van Tassel RA, et al. Left atrial appendage obliteration: mechanisms of healing and intracardiac integration. JACC Cardiovasc Interv 2010;3(8):870–7.

30. Holmes DR, Reddy VY, Turi ZG, et al. Percutaneous closure of the left atrial appendage versus warfarin therapy for prevention of stroke in patients with atrial fibrillation: a randomised non-inferiority trial. Lancet 2009;374(9689):534–42.

31. Holmes DR Jr, Kar S, Price MJ, et al. Prospective randomized evaluation of the Watchman Left Atrial Appendage Closure device in patients with atrial fibrillation versus long-term warfarin therapy: the PREVAIL trial. J Am Coll Cardiol 2014;64(1):1–12.

32. Waksman R, Pendyala LK. Overview of the Food and Drug Administration circulatory system devices panel meetings on WATCHMAN left atrial appendage closure therapy. Am J Cardiol 2015; 115(3):378–84.

33. Boersma LV, Ince H, Kische S, et al. Efficacy and safety of left atrial appendage closure with WATCHMAN in patients with or without contraindication to oral anticoagulation: 1-Year follow-up outcome data of the EWOLUTION trial. Heart Rhythm 2017;14(9):1302–8.

34. Boersma LV, Ince H, Kische S, et al. Evaluating Real-world clinical outcomes in atrial fibrillation patients receiving the WATCHMAN left atrial appendage closure technology. Circ Arrhythm Electrophysiol 2019;12(4):e006841.

35. Boersma LV, Schmidt B, Betts TR, et al. Implant success and safety of left atrial appendage closure with the WATCHMAN device: peri-procedural outcomes from the EWOLUTION registry. Eur Heart J 2016; 37(31):2465–74.

36. Holmes DR Jr, Doshi SK, Kar S, et al. Left atrial appendage closure as an alternative to warfarin for stroke prevention in atrial fibrillation: a patient-level meta-analysis. J Am Coll Cardiol 2015;65(24): 2614–23.

37. Reddy VY, Doshi SK, Kar S, et al. 5-Year outcomes after left atrial appendage closure: from the PREVAIL and PROTECT AF trials. J Am Coll Cardiol 2017;70(24):2964–75.

38. Reddy VY, Gibson DN, Kar S, et al. Post-approval U.S. experience with left atrial appendage closure for stroke prevention in atrial fibrillation. J Am Coll Cardiol 2017;69(3):253–61.

39. Reddy VY, Holmes D, Doshi SK, et al. Safety of percutaneous left atrial appendage closure: results from the watchman left atrial appendage system for embolic protection in patients with AF (PROTECT AF) clinical trial and the continued access registry. Circulation 2011;123(4):417–24.

40. Reddy VY, Mobius-Winkler S, Miller MA, et al. Left atrial appendage closure with the watchman device in patients with a contraindication for oral anticoagulation: the ASAP study (ASA Plavix feasibility study with watchman left atrial appendage closure technology). J Am Coll Cardiol 2013;61(25):2551–6.

41. Varosy P, Masoudi F, Reisman M, et al. Procedural safety of WATCHMAN implantation: the US nested post approval study. J Am Coll Cardiol 2018.

42. Phillips KP, Walker DT, Humphries JA. Combined catheter ablation for atrial fibrillation and Watchman(R) left atrial appendage occlusion procedures: five-year experience. J Arrhythm 2016;32(2):119–26.

43. Fauchier L, Cinaud A, Brigadeau F, et al. Device-related thrombosis after percutaneous left atrial appendage occlusion for atrial fibrillation. J Am Coll Cardiol 2018;71(14):1528–36.

44. Kubo S, Mizutani Y, Meemook K, et al. Incidence, characteristics, and clinical course of device-related thrombus after watchman left atrial appendage occlusion device implantation in atrial fibrillation patients. JACC Clin Electrophysiol 2017; 3(12):1380–6.

45. Pracon R, Bangalore S, Dzielinska Z, et al. Device thrombosis after percutaneous left atrial appendage occlusion is related to patient and procedural characteristics but not to duration of postimplantation dual antiplatelet therapy. Circ Cardiovasc Interv 2018;11(3):e005997.

46. Shamim S, Magalski A, Chhatriwalla AK, et al. Transesophageal echocardiographic diagnosis of a WATCHMAN left atrial appendage closure device thrombus 10 years following implantation. Echocardiography 2017;34(1):128–30.

47. Landmesser U, Tondo C, Camm J, et al. Left atrial appendage occlusion with the AMPLATZER Amulet device: one-year follow-up from the prospective global Amulet observational registry. EuroIntervention 2018;14(5):e590–7.

48. Tzikas A, Shakir S, Gafoor S, et al. Left atrial appendage occlusion for stroke prevention in atrial fibrillation: multicentre experience with the AMPLATZER Cardiac Plug. EuroIntervention 2016;11(10): 1170–9.

49. Nielsen-Kudsk JE, Johnsen SP, Wester P, et al. Left atrial appendage occlusion versus standard medical care in patients with atrial fibrillation and intracerebral haemorrhage: a propensity score-matched follow-up study. EuroIntervention 2017; 13(3):371–8.

50. Hijazi ZM, SJ. Nonpharmacologic therapy to prevent embolization in patients with atrial fibrillation. UpTo Date; 2019. Available at: https://www.uptodate.com/contents/nonpharmacologic-therapy-to-prevent-embolization-in-patients-with-atrial-fibrillation?search=nonpharmacologic%20therapy%20to%20prevent%20embolization%20in%20patients%20with%20atrial%20fibrillation&source=search_result&selectedTitle=1~150&usage_type=default&display_rank=1. Accessed December 19, 2019.

Thromboembolism in Atrial Fibrillation
Role of the Left Atrial Appendage

Payam Safavi-Naeini, MD[a,1], Abdi Rasekh, MD[b,c],*

KEYWORDS

- Atrial fibrillation • AF-related stroke • Left atrial appendage • AF-related thromboembolism

KEY POINTS

- Atrial fibrillation (AF) increases the risk of ischemic stroke by 4-fold to 5-fold. The annual rate of AF-related stroke is 5%.
- Approximately 80% of embolism-related deaths are from AF-related stroke and 20% from AF-related thromboembolism of limbs and visceral arteries.
- The left atrial appendage (LAA) is the main site of thrombus formation in patients with nonvalvular AF (>90%) and valvular AF (57%).
- LAA function and morphology have significant roles in predicting the propensity of thrombus formation in patients with AF.

INTRODUCTION

Atrial fibrillation (AF) is the most common sustained cardiac arrhythmia, with a prevalence of 1% to 2% in the general population.[1] The prevalence of AF increases with age, ranging from 0.1% in people younger than 50 years, 5.9% in those older than 65 years, and 10% in individuals aged 75 years or older.[2] An estimated 2.7 to 6.1 million people in the United States and around 8 million people in the European Union have AF. Because of aging populations, the prevalence of AF is expected to be more than 12 million in the United States, and 14 to 17 million in the European Union by 2030.[3,4]

AF is associated with substantial morbidity and mortality, especially caused by atrial thrombus formation and peripheral embolization. More than 750,000 hospitalizations and an estimated 130,000 deaths occur each year caused by AF.

The average medical costs for patients with AF is about $8705 higher per year than for people without AF, costing the United States about $6 billion each year.[5] AF-related thromboembolism usually manifests in the brain, which is extremely vulnerable to ischemia, but also can cause complications in other organ systems, such as acute renal thromboembolism and acute thromboembolic mesenteric ischemia.[6] Approximately 80% of embolism-related deaths are from AF-related stroke and 20% from AF-related thromboembolism of limbs and visceral arteries.[6] AF is diagnosed in 60% to 95% of patients with acute limb ischemia, 31% in patients with splenic artery embolization, 55% in patients with acute renal ischemia, and 47% in patients with mesenteric ischemia.[7] A Danish population study among patients with a hospital diagnosis showed that AF increased risk of peripheral thromboembolic events (relative risk [RR] 4.0, 95% confidence

a Electrophysiology Clinical Research and Innovation, Texas Heart Institute, Houston, TX, USA; b Cardiology, Baylor College of Medicine, 6624 Fannin Street Suite 2480, Houston, TX 77030, USA; c Cardiology, Texas Heart Institute, Houston, TX, USA
1 Present address: 2425 Augusta Drive Apartment 63, Houston, TX 77057.
* Corresponding author. Cardiology, Baylor College of Medicine, 6624 Fannin Street Suite 2480, Houston, TX 77030.
E-mail address: arasekh@bcm.edu

Card Electrophysiol Clin 12 (2020) 13–20
https://doi.org/10.1016/j.ccep.2019.11.003
1877-9182/20/© 2019 Elsevier Inc. All rights reserved.

cardiacEP.theclinics.com

interval [CI] 3.5–4.6 in men; and RR 5.7, 95% CI 5.1–6.3 in women).[8]

THROMBOEMBOLISM IN ATRIAL FIBRILLATION
Ischemic Stroke

The most clinically noticeable and serious thromboembolic event in patients with AF is ischemic stroke.[9] AF increases the risk of ischemic stroke by 4 to 5 times. The annual rate of AF-related stroke is 5%, which accounts for greater than or equal to 15% of all strokes in the United States, 36% of strokes for people aged more than 80 years, and up to 20% that are cryptogenic strokes. The incidence of AF-related stroke increases with age, from about 1.3% in patients between 50 and 59 years old, to 5.1% in patients between 80 and 89 years old.[10] Patients with paroxysmal AF have almost the same risk for stroke as individuals with persistent or long-standing persistent AF.[11]

AF-related strokes are associated with increased risk of stroke severity, permanent disability, and greater short-term and long-term mortality, and patients with AF-related stroke have 2 times the risk of mortality and 3 times the risk of stroke recurrence within 1 year compared with patients without AF.[12]

Splenic Artery Embolization

Splenic thromboembolic infarction is a rare cause of acute abdominal pain. The annual incidence of AF-related acute mesenteric ischemia is 0.14% with 70% lethality at 12 months.[6] Cardiogenic splenic emboli account for 22% to 55% of all causes of splenic infarction.[13] A 10-year retrospective study[14] to examine the risk factors of splenic infarction showed that AF was the most common risk factors for thrombosis (11 out of 48 patients [23%] had AF). Previous cardiac valvular surgery, previous thromboembolism, significant hematologic disease, malignancy, oral contraceptives, antiphospholipid syndrome, and severe liver disease were other risk factors of splenic infarction.

Acute Renal Thromboembolism

Acute renal embolus is a rare cause of acute kidney injury. Renal embolism most often originated from the heart because of AF. In a study of 62 patients with acute renal infarction (ARI), 30 patients (48%) had embolic ARI with a cardiac origin. The prevalence of AF was 70% among these patients (21 out of 30).[15]

In another retrospective study of 67 patients with renal infarction by Rhee and colleagues,[16] AF was the most common cause of acute renal ischemia (detected in 17 cases [25.4%]), followed by direct vessel injury (22.4%) and hypercoagulable state, including protein C and S deficiency, malignancy, and bedridden state (20.9%).

Atrial Fibrillation–Related Mesenteric Artery Embolization

Acute mesenteric ischemia is an uncommon disease (estimated between 0.09% and 0.2% of all acute surgical admissions) with a high mortality.[17]

Approximately 50% of all cases of acute mesenteric ischemia are caused by acute mesenteric embolism.[18] Acute mesenteric embolism most commonly has a cardiac origin and about 50% of patients have AF.[19,20]

Atrial Fibrillation–Related Peripheral Arterial Disease

Many different studies showed that patients with AF have a higher risk of peripheral arterial disease (PAD) and, conversely, PAD independently increases the risk of AF.[21] In the years 2000 to 2001, a longitudinal, nationwide, population-based study among 3814 patients with AF and 15,364 patients without AF from Taiwan National Health Insurance Research Database showed that AF was associated with a significantly higher risk of PAD (adjusted hazard ratio, 1.58; 95% CI, 1.32–1.88).[22]

MECHANISMS OF THROMBOEMBOLISM IN ATRIAL FIBRILLATION

Left atrial thrombi are found in up to 14% of patients in whom AF lasts more than 2 days by transesophageal echocardiography (TEE); thrombi size ranges between 0.2 and 4.2 cm.[23] In addition, there is a small but significant chance of LA thrombus formation despite oral anticoagulation treatment in patients with AF. TEE revealed LA thrombus in 1.6% of patients treated with warfarin for at least 6 months.[24] Most often, thromboembolism occurs during episodes of AF, or in the first 10 days after conversion to sinus rhythm.[25] AF is characterized by disorganized electrical activity in the atria, resulting in ineffective irregular contraction and incomplete ejection of blood from the atria into the ventricles and stasis of blood, especially within the left atrial appendage (LAA), which is the main source of thrombus formation in patients with AF. The LAA is the main site of thrombus formation in AF, and more than 90% of the thrombi found in patients with nonvalvular AF and 57% found in valvular AF are formed in the LAA.[26]

Beside blood stasis in the LAA, other components of the Virchow's triad, such as structural heart disease with endocardial damage and hypercoagulable state (caused by abnormalities in platelet and hemostatic variables) play roles in thrombogenic tendency among patients with AF.[27] AF results in increased platelet activation (detected by increasing platelet P-selectin) and thrombin generation (detected by increasing thrombin-antithrombin complex) especially in circulation and to a greater extent in LA. In addition, AF leads to endothelial dysfunction (detected by increasing asymmetric dimethylarginine) and inflammation (detected by increasing soluble cluster of differentiation 40 [CD40] ligand).[28] Patients with AF have more than 2-fold higher circulating levels of CRP (a marker of systemic inflammation) compared with those without AF, and CRP level increase is more prominent in persistent AF compared with paroxysmal AF.[29] Some small studies showed that systemic inflammation has a significant role in thromboembolism among patients with AF.[30] In a study that included patients with AF enrolled in the Apixaban for Reduction in Stroke and Other Thromboembolic Events in Atrial Fibrillation (ARISTOTLE) trial for incident strokes, interleukin 6 (IL-6) and CRP were analyzed among 14,954 patients with a median follow-up of 1.9 years.[31] In patients with AF treated with anticoagulants, high-sensitivity CRP and IL-6 had significant associations with all-cause mortality but they did not show significant associations with the risk of stroke or major bleeding.

The incidence of AF-related stroke varies widely among patients with AF, ranging from 1% to 20% per year.[32] Patients with chronic AF frequently have LAA remodeling, including dilatation (a 3-fold increase in LAA volume), stretching, reduction in pectinate muscle volume, and endocardial fibroelastosis.[33] LAA function and morphology have significant roles in predicting the propensity of thrombus formation in patients with AF.

LEFT ATRIAL APPENDAGE ANATOMY AND RISK FOR STROKE
Embryology and Anatomy of the Left Atrial Appendage

The LAA is derived from the original embryonic left atrium (LA), unlike the rest of the LA, which is formed from pulmonary veins; LAA starts to develop in the third week of pregnancy.[34] The LAA is a long, trabeculated cul-de-sac with a narrow neck and lobulated end, which lies in the left atrioventricular groove in proximity to the left circumflex artery, left superior pulmonary

vein posteriorly, the mitral valve annulus, and the left phrenic nerve.[35] Both parasympathetic and sympathetic fibers richly innervate the LAA. Alongside the atria (main sources of atrial natriuretic peptide [ANP]) and ventricles (main sources of brain natriuretic peptide [BNP]), the LAA also secretes ANP and BNP. Both ANP and BNP promote vasodilation, diuresis, and natriuresis in response to atrial and ventricular volume/pressure expansion.[36] Although the ventricles are the main source of BNP, the atria become the prominent source of BNP in AF.[37] The endocardium of the LAA contains pectinate muscles; there are 3 regions of the LAA: the ostium, the neck, and the lobar regions.[38] There are also lobes[39] (Fig. 1).

The most common shape of the LAA ostium is elliptical (68.9%), with a short diameter ranging from 12 to 39 mm, long diameter ranging from 25 to 86 mm, and a depth ranging from 16 to 51 mm. The less common shapes of ostium are round, triangular, water drop–like, and footlike.[40] Anatomic studies described different shapes of the LAA as a long, narrow, tubular, wavy, or hooked appendage with a narrow junction and crenelated lumen.[41] Developmental abnormalities of the LAA are rare, including a congenital absence of the LAA, isomerism of the LAA, giant LAA, and congenital LAA aneurysm.[40] Congenital LAA aneurysms are associated with potentially serious complications, such as life-threatening systemic thromboembolism, supraventricular arrhythmias, and cardiac dysfunction.[42]

Number of Left Atrial Appendage Lobes

A study of 500 normal autopsy hearts showed that the 2-lobe LAA is the most frequent type of LAA (54%), followed by 3 lobes (23%), 1 lobe (20%), and 4 lobes (3%.27). There are no significant age-related or sex-related differences in LAA morphologies.[43] The number of LAA lobes is an independent risk factor for LAA thrombus (odds ratio [OR], 2.469; 95% CI, 1.495–4.078; $P<.001$). A prospective study among 633 patients showed that most patients with LAA thrombus (32 out of 34, 94.4%) had 3 or more LAA lobes and LAA thrombus was only observed in 2 (0.7%) of 296 patients with fewer than 3 lobes.[44] In another study among 472 consecutive patients with nonvalvular AF, the left atrial thrombus (LAT) incidence rate increased from a single lobe to multiple lobes, and the number of LAA lobes was an independent predictor of LAT (single, double, multiple, OR, 2.37; 95% CI, 1.37–4.09; $P = .002$).[45]

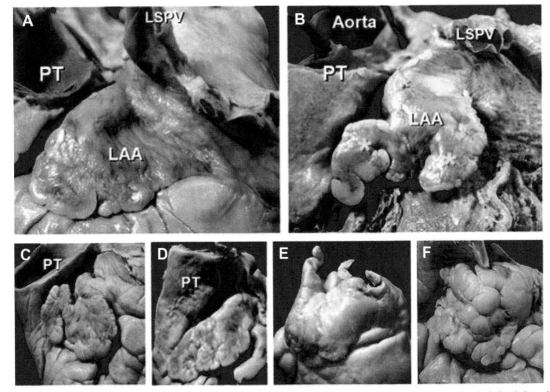

Fig. 1. Anatomic variants of LAA. (*A, B*) The different morphologies of the LAA, including a single lobe (*A*) and multilobed (*B, asterisks*). (*C–F*) The common variants of LAA morphology: chicken wing (*C*), windsock (*D*), cactus (*E*), and cauliflower (*F*). LSPV, left superior pulmonary vein; PT, pulmonary trunk. (*From* Cabrera JA, Saremi F, Sánchez-Quintana D. Left atrial appendage: anatomy and imaging landmarks pertinent to percutaneous transcatheter occlusion. Heart 2014;100:1636; with permission.)

The Left Atrial Appendage Size and Trabeculation

Beinart and colleagues[46] studied 144 patients with nonvalvular AF who were not receiving warfarin, and who underwent MRI/magnetic resonance angiography before the AF ablation procedure. The mean LAA volume was 15.5 ± 7.9 cm^3 (95% CI, 14.2–16.8) and the mean LAA depth was 3.28 ± 0.8 cm (95% CI, 3.14–3.41). The LAA volume, LAA depth, and LAA neck dimensions were larger in patients with sustained stroke/transient ischemic attack (TIA) compared with patients without a history of embolic events. An LAA morphologic study of 678 patients who were referred for AF ablation with computed tomography images by Khurram and colleagues[47] showed that extensive LAA trabeculations and smaller LAA orifice size are independent risk factors for TIA/stroke in patients with AF.

In a study among 1224 patients, researchers showed that the left atrial volume index (LAVI) is greater in patients with cardioembolic (CE) stroke compared with patients with non-CE stroke (41.4 ± 18.0 mL/m^2 vs 28.6 ± 12.2 mL/m^2;

$P<.001$). In addition, LAVI was associated with detection of AF in patients with embolic stroke of undetermined source.[48]

The Left Atrial Appendage Shape

In the past, TEE was the main tool to evaluate LAA morphology, but advancements in cardiac computed tomography and cardiac magnetic resonance have enabled more comprehensive studies of LAA morphology. The LAA morphology is generally classified into 4 types, known as chicken wing, cauliflower, cactus, and windsock[49] (see **Fig. 1**). The chicken wing is characterized by having a dominant central lobe with a sharp bend in the proximal or middle part of it or folding back of the LAA anatomy on itself at some distance from the perceived LAA ostium. The cactus has a dominant central lobe with secondary lobes extending from above and below the central lobe. The windsock has 1 main lobe and other smaller lobes arising from the dominant lobe in an inferior direction. The cauliflower has a shorter length than the others and more complex internal structures.[49] In a study among 932 patients with drug-refractory

AF using cardiac computed tomography and cardiac magnetic resonance, patients with chicken-wing LAA morphology had the least prevalence of embolic events (4%) and the cauliflower LAA morphology had the highest prevalence of embolic events (18%).[50]

In a recent study, researchers hypothesized that severe or acute angle bend in the proximal or middle lobe is responsible for protection against stroke risk in the chicken-wing morphology, so the chicken-wing LAA morphology with a greater than 90° bend has a similar risk of stroke as a non–chicken-wing LAA.[51] LAA morphology was classified into 2 groups, based on the angle between the orifice and the LAA. Low-risk LAA morphology (LAA-L) was defined as a bend or fold with an acute angle (<90°) at the proximal or middle portion of the LAA, and high-risk morphology (LAA-H) was described as all other shapes. Patients in the LAA-H group had a higher risk for CE stroke (OR, 5.4; 95% CI, 2.1–13.7; $P<.001$) and embolic stroke of unknown source (ESUS) (OR, 2.78; 95% CI, 1.2–6.4; $P = .016$). When patients were classified into 3 groups (chicken wing/LAA-L, chicken wing/LAA-H, and non–chicken wing/LAA-H), the prevalences of CE stroke and ESUS were similar in non–chicken-wing/LAA-H and chicken-wing/LAA-H groups and was higher compared with the chicken-wing/LAA-L group (CE 39.2%, 39.1% vs 34.4%; ESUS 38.2%, 36.2% vs 25%).

Atrial Tissue Remodeling and Left Atrial Appendage Thrombus

A study among 178 patients with AF[52] undergoing TEE and late gadolinium enhancement MRI (LGE-MRI) before cardioversion or ablation procedure showed that patients with left atrial fibrosis greater than 20% had a higher chance of having an LAA thrombus (OR, 4.6; $P = .02$).

LEFT ATRIAL APPENDAGE PHYSIOLOGY AND RISK FOR STROKE

The hemodynamic function of the LAA is another risk factor for thrombus formation, and both poor appendage contraction and dilatation increase risks of thrombosis.[53]

Although LAA has been largely considered to be nonfunctional, it is an actively contracting structure and TEE studies showed contractile activities of LAA by visualizing flow velocity waveforms on pulsed Doppler echocardiography of LAA. Three LAA Doppler flow patterns have been described by TEE color Doppler.[54]

Type I is observed in sinus rhythm, characterized by a biphasic pattern (waves of filling and emptying), with mean peak velocities of 28 ± 12 cm/s for filling waves and 31 ± 9 cm/s for emptying waves. Type II is observed in patients with AF with dilated LAA (LAA area 421 ± 40 mm^2), characterized by a sawtooth emptying pattern, with a mean peak velocity of 49 ± 12 cm/s. Type III is observed in patients with AF with very dilated LAAs (LAA area 619 ± 96 mm^2), characterized by the absence of any active emptying pattern.

This study showed that absence of or very low LAA Doppler flow (type III) has a strong correlation with thrombus formation (6 patients out of 7 with thrombus had type III pattern).

In a study among 57 patients with AF who presented to the neurology service for evaluation of stroke or TIA, peak positive LA strain and strain rate were measured during left ventricle (LV) systole, and peak negative strain and strain rate were measured at LV end-diastole or during LA contraction. Patients with stroke had reduced peak negative (-3.2% ± 1.2% vs -6.9% ± 4.2%, $P<.001$) and peak positive (14% ± 11% vs 25% ± 12%, $P<.001$) LA strain values compared with controls.[55] In another study using tissue Doppler imaging with TEE and transthoracic echocardiography to measure LAA contraction velocity among 141 patients, Uretsky and colleagues[56] showed that LAA contraction velocity was lower in patients with AF and history of stroke/TIA compared with patients with AF without history of stroke/TIA (11 ± 3 cm/s vs 15 ± 6 cm/s, $P = .008$). Almost one-third of patients with an LAA flow velocity less than or equal to 11 cm/s had LAA thrombus.

RELATIONSHIP BETWEEN THE DEMOGRAPHIC, CLINICAL, LABORATORY, AND ECHOCARDIOGRAPHIC CHARACTERISTICS OF PATIENTS WITH ATRIAL FIBRILLATION AND RISK OF STROKE

Congestive heart failure (CHF) (RR 1.4), hypertension (RR 1.6), older age (RR 1.4 per decade), diabetes (RR 1.7), history of prior stroke/TIA (RR 2.5), coronary artery disease (RR 1.5), and female sex (RR 1.31) are strong independent predictors of stroke in patients with AF.[57] Moreover, a meta-analysis of 538,479 patients and 41,719 incident thromboembolic events from 18 studies showed that patients with estimated glomerular filtration rate (eGFR) less than 60 mL/min compared with those with eGFR greater than or equal to 60 mL/min had an increased risk for developing thromboembolic events (RR, 1.62; 95% CI, 1.40–1.87; $P<.001$]). In a study among patients with AF who had acute cerebrovascular ischemic events during treatment with novel,

Table-1
Left atrial appendage and atrial fibrillation–related thromboembolic events

LAA Parameter	Findings
Number of LAA lobes	Higher number of LAA lobes increases risk of LAA thrombus[43]
The LAA size and trabeculation	The larger LAA volume, LAA depth, and LAA neck dimensions increase risk of stroke/TIA[46] The extensive LAA trabeculations and smaller LAA orifice size increase risk of stroke/TIA[47]
The LAA shape	Patients with chicken-wing LAA morphology are less likely to develop embolic events[50] The chicken wing is characterized by having a sharp bend in the proximal or middle part of the dominant lobe
Atrial tissue remodeling and LAA thrombus	Patients with left atrial fibrosis > 20% had a higher chance of having an LAA thrombus[52]
LAA blood flow velocity	Low LAA contraction velocity is a risk factor for LAA thrombus[56]

including non–vitamin K antagonists, oral anticoagulants (NOACs), patients treated with off-label low-dose NOACs and patients with atrial enlargement had a higher risk of ischemic events (OR, 3.18; 95% CI, 1.95–5.85; P = .0001; and OR, 6.64; 95% CI, 4.63–9.52, P = .0001, respectively). In addition, a high CHA_2DS_2-VASc (congestive heart failure; hypertension; age $\geq$75 years; diabetes mellitus; prior stroke, TIA, or thromboembolism; vascular disease; age 65–74 years; sex category) score was associated with increased risk of cerebrovascular events (OR, 1.72 for each point increase; 95% CI, 1.58–1.88; P = .0001).[58]

CHA_2DS_2-VASc scoring system is used to assess the risk of thromboembolism in patients with AF. The maximum number of this score is 9. CHF, hypertension, diabetes mellitus, vascular disease, age between 65 and 74 years, and female sex have 1 point. Prior stroke or TIA or thromboembolism, and age greater than or equal to 75 years have 2 points. The European Society of Cardiology (ESC) guidelines recommend using oral anticoagulation in men with a score of 1 or higher and women with a score of 2 or higher.[59] Recent studies suggested that female sex is a risk modifier and is age dependent, and adding female sex to the CHA_2DS_2-VASc score matters among patients with age greater than 65 years or having greater than or equal to 2 non–sex-related stroke risk factors.[60] Accordingly, the optimal risk score is still in evolution.

SUMMARY

The LA has a prominent role in AF-related thromboembolic events. Beside the clinical comorbidities, LAA anatomy and physiology have significant roles in predicting the propensity for thrombus formation in patients with AF (**Table 1**).

DISCLOSURE

No conflict of interest.

REFERENCES

1. Malladi V, Naeini PS, Razavi M, et al. Endovascular ablation of atrial fibrillation. Anesthesiology 2014; 120:1513–9.
2. Safavi Naeini P, Rasekh A. A review of clinical trials on LARIAT device. J Atrial Fibrillation 2015;8:1317.
3. Passman R, Bernstein RA. New appraisal of atrial fibrillation burden and stroke prevention. Stroke 2016;47:570–6.
4. Zoni-Berisso M, Lercari F, Carazza T, et al. Epidemiology of atrial fibrillation: European perspective. Clin Epidemiol 2014;6:213–20.
5. Mozaffarian D, Benjamin Emelia J, Go Alan S, et al. Heart disease and stroke statistics—2015 update. Circulation 2015;131:e29–322.
6. Menke J, Luthje L, Kastrup A, et al. Thromboembolism in atrial fibrillation. Am J Cardiol 2010;105: 502–10.
7. Wasilewska M, Gosk-Bierska I. Thromboembolism associated with atrial fibrillation as a cause of limb and organ ischemia. Adv Clin Exp Med 2013;22: 865–73.
8. Frost L, Engholm G, Johnsen S, et al. Incident thromboembolism in the aorta and the renal, mesenteric, pelvic, and extremity arteries after discharge from the hospital with a diagnosis of atrial fibrillation. Arch Intern Med 2001;161:272–6.

9. Sharma M, Khalighi K. Non-pharmacologic approach to prevent embolization in patients with atrial fibrillation in whom anticoagulation is contraindicated. Clin Pract 2017;7:898.

10. Jonas DE, Kahwati LC, Yun JDY, et al. Screening for atrial fibrillation with electrocardiography: evidence report and systematic review for the US preventive services task Force. JAMA 2018;320:485–98.

11. Safavi-Naeini P, Rasekh A. Closure of left atrial appendage to prevent stroke: devices and status. Tex Heart Inst J 2018;45:172–4.

12. Safavi-Naeini P, Razavi M, Saeed M, et al. A review of the LARIAT suture delivery device for left atrial appendage closure. J Tehran Heart Cent 2015;10: 69–73.

13. Chiu C-CW, Chiung Z. Atrial fibrillation and splenic infarction presenting with unexplained fever and persistent abdominal pain a case report and review of the literature. Acta Cardiol Sin 2012.

14. Antopolsky M, Hiller N, Salameh S, et al. Splenic infarction: 10 years of experience. Am J Emerg Med 2009;27:262–5.

15. Caravaca-Fontán F, Pampa Saico S, Elías Triviño S, et al. Acute renal infarction: clinical characteristics and prognostic factors. Nefrología 2016;36:141–8.

16. Rhee H, Song SH, Won Lee D, et al. The significance of clinical features in the prognosis of acute renal infarction: single center experience. Clin Exp Nephrol 2012;16:611–6.

17. Bala M, Kashuk J, Moore EE, et al. Acute mesenteric ischemia: guidelines of the World Society of Emergency surgery. World J Emerg Surg 2017;12:38.

18. Acosta S, Ögren M, Sternby N-H, et al. Fatal nonocclusive mesenteric ischaemia: population-based incidence and risk factors. J Intern Med 2006;259: 305–13.

19. Björck M, Koelemay M, Acosta S, et al. Editor's choice – management of the diseases of mesenteric arteries and veins: clinical practice guidelines of the European Society of Vascular Surgery (ESVS). Eur J Vasc Endovasc Surg 2017;53:460–510.

20. Park WM, Gloviczki P, Cherry KJ Jr, et al. Contemporary management of acute mesenteric ischemia: factors associated with survival. J Vasc Surg 2002; 35:445–52.

21. Proietti M. Is there a relationship between atrial fibrillation and peripheral arterial disease. e-Journal of Cardiology Practice 2018;16.

22. Chang C-J, Chen Y-T, Liu C-S, et al. Atrial fibrillation increases the risk of peripheral arterial disease with relative complications and mortality: a population-based cohort study. Medicine (Baltimore) 2016;95: e3002.

23. Thambidorai SK, Murray RD, Parakh K, et al. Utility of transesophageal echocardiography in identification of thrombogenic milieu in patients with atrial fibrillation (an ACUTE ancillary study). Am J Cardiol 2005;96:935–41.

24. Scherr D, Dalal D, Chilukuri K, et al. Incidence and predictors of left atrial thrombus prior to catheter ablation of atrial fibrillation. J Cardiovasc Electrophysiol 2009;20:379–84.

25. Wakai A, O'Neill JO. Emergency management of atrial fibrillation. Postgrad Med J 2003;79:313–9.

26. Blackshear JL, Odell JA. Appendage obliteration to reduce stroke in cardiac surgical patients with atrial fibrillation. Ann Thorac Surg 1996;61:755–9.

27. Watson T, Shantsila E, Lip GY. Mechanisms of thrombogenesis in atrial fibrillation: Virchow's triad revisited. Lancet 2009;373:155–66.

28. Lim HS, Willoughby SR, Schultz C, et al. Effect of atrial fibrillation on atrial thrombogenesis in humans: impact of rate and rhythm. J Am Coll Cardiol 2013; 61:852–60.

29. Chung Mina K, Martin David O, Sprecher D, et al. C-Reactive protein elevation in patients with atrial arrhythmias. Circulation 2001;104:2886–91.

30. Boos CJ, Anderson RA, Lip GYH. Is atrial fibrillation an inflammatory disorder? Eur Heart J 2005;27: 136–49.

31. Hijazi Z, Aulin J, Andersson U, et al. Biomarkers of inflammation and risk of cardiovascular events in anticoagulated patients with atrial fibrillation. Heart 2016;102:508.

32. Furie Karen L, Goldstein Larry B, Albers Gregory W, et al. Oral antithrombotic agents for the prevention of stroke in nonvalvular atrial fibrillation. Stroke 2012; 43:3442–53.

33. Shirani J, Alaeddini J. Structural remodeling of the left atrial appendage in patients with chronic nonvalvular atrial fibrillation: implications for thrombus formation, systemic embolism, and assessment by transesophageal echocardiography. Cardiovasc Pathol 2000;9:95–101.

34. Al-Saady NM, Obel OA, Camm AJ. Left atrial appendage: structure, function, and role in thromboembolism. Heart 1999;82:547–54.

35. Patti G, Pengo V, Marcucci R, et al. The left atrial appendage: from embryology to prevention of thromboembolism. Eur Heart J 2017;38:877–87.

36. Wilber DJ. Neurohormonal regulation and the left atrial appendage. J Am Coll Cardiol 2018;71:145.

37. Luchner A, Stevens TL, Borgeson DD, et al. Differential atrial and ventricular expression of myocardial BNP during evolution of heart failure. Am J Physiol 1998;274:H1684–9.

38. Barbero U, Ho SY. Anatomy of the atria: a road map to the left atrial appendage. Herzschrittmacherther Elektrophysiol 2017;347–54.

39. Cabrera JA, Saremi F, Sánchez-Quintana D. Left atrial appendage: anatomy and imaging landmarks pertinent to percutaneous transcatheter occlusion. Heart 2014;100:1636.

40. Naksuk N, Padmanabhan D, Yogeswaran V, et al. Left atrial appendage: embryology, anatomy, physiology, arrhythmia and therapeutic intervention. JACC Clin Electrophysiol 2016;2:403–12.

41. Regazzoli D, Ancona F, Trevisi N, et al. Left atrial appendage: physiology, pathology, and role as a therapeutic target. Biomed Res Int 2015;2015:13.

42. Chen Y, Mou Y, Jiang L-J, et al. Congenital giant left atrial appendage aneurysm: a case report. J Cardiothorac Surg 2017;12:15.

43. Veinot John P, Harrity Phillip J, Gentile F, et al. Anatomy of the normal left atrial appendage. Circulation 1997;96:3112–5.

44. Yamamoto M, Seo Y, Kawamatsu N, et al. Complex left atrial appendage morphology and left atrial appendage thrombus formation in patients with atrial fibrillation. Circ Cardiovasc Imaging 2014;7:337–43.

45. Wang F, Zhu M, Wang X, et al. Predictive value of left atrial appendage lobes on left atrial thrombus or spontaneous echo contrast in patients with non-valvular atrial fibrillation. BMC Cardiovasc Disord 2018;18(1):153.

46. Beinart R, Heist EK, Newell JB, et al. Left atrial appendage dimensions predict the risk of stroke/TIA in patients with atrial fibrillation. J Cardiovasc Electrophysiol 2011;22:10–5.

47. Khurram IM, Dewire J, Mager M, et al. Relationship between left atrial appendage morphology and stroke in patients with atrial fibrillation. Heart Rhythm 2013;10:1843–9.

48. Jordan K, Yaghi S, Poppas A, et al. Left atrial volume index is associated with cardioembolic stroke and atrial fibrillation detection after embolic stroke of undetermined source. Stroke 2019;50:1997–2001.

49. Wang Y, Di Biase L, Horton RP, et al. Left atrial appendage studied by computed tomography to help planning for appendage closure device placement. J Cardiovasc Electrophysiol 2010;21:973–82.

50. Di Biase L, Santangeli P, Anselmino M, et al. Does the left atrial appendage morphology correlate with the risk of stroke in patients with atrial fibrillation?: Results from a multicenter study. J Am Coll Cardiol 2012;60:531–8.

51. Yaghi S, Chang A, Akiki R, et al. The left atrial appendage morphology is associated with embolic stroke subtypes using a simple classification system: a proof of concept study. J Cardiovasc Comput Tomogr 2019 [pii:S1934–5925(19)30071-1]: undefined-undefined.

52. Akoum N, Fernandez G, Wilson B, et al. Association of atrial fibrosis quantified using LGE-MRI with atrial appendage thrombus and spontaneous contrast on transesophageal echocardiography in patients with atrial fibrillation. J Cardiovasc Electrophysiol 2013;24:1104–9.

53. Kortz RAM, Delemarre BJ, van Dantzig JM, et al. Left atrial appendage blood flow determined by transesophageal echocardiography in healthy subjects. Am J Cardiol 1993;71:976–81.

54. Garcia-Fernandez MA, Torrecilla EG, San Roman D, et al. Left atrial appendage Doppler flow patterns: implications on thrombus formation. Am Heart J 1992;124:955–61.

55. Azemi T, Rabdiya VM, Ayirala SR, et al. Left atrial strain is reduced in patients with atrial fibrillation, stroke or TIA, and low risk CHADS2 Scores. J Am Soc Echocardiogr 2012;25:1327–32.

56. Uretsky S, Shah A, Bangalore S, et al. Assessment of left atrial appendage function with transthoracic tissue Doppler echocardiography. Eur J Echocardiogr 2009;10:363–71.

57. Fuster V, Rydén Lars E, Cannom David S, et al. ACC/AHA/ESC 2006 guidelines for the management of patients with atrial fibrillation. Circulation 2006;114:e257–354.

58. Paciaroni M, Agnelli G, Caso V, et al. Causes and risk factors of cerebral ischemic events in patients with atrial fibrillation treated with non–Vitamin k antagonist oral anticoagulants for stroke prevention. Stroke 2019;50:2168–74.

59. Kirchhof P, Benussi S, Kotecha D, et al. 2016 ESC guidelines for the management of atrial fibrillation developed in collaboration with EACTS. Eur J Cardiothorac Surg 2016;50:e1–88.

60. January Craig T, Wann LS, Calkins H, et al. 2019 AHA/ACC/HRS focused update of the 2014 AHA/ACC/HRS guideline for the management of patients with atrial fibrillation: a report of the American College of Cardiology/American Heart Association Task Force on clinical practice guidelines and the Heart Rhythm Society in Collaboration with the Society of Thoracic Surgeons. Circulation 2019;140:e125–51.

Role of the Left Atrial Appendage in Systemic Homeostasis, Arrhythmogenesis, and Beyond

Ghulam Murtaza, MD[a], Bharath Yarlagadda, MD[b], Krishna Akella, DO[a],
Domenico G. Della Rocca, MD[c,d], Rakesh Gopinathannair, MD[a],
Andrea Natale, MD[c,d], Dhanunjaya Lakkireddy, MD, FHRS[a,*]

KEYWORDS

- Left atrial appendage • Systemic homeostasis • Arrhythmogenesis

KEY POINTS

- Left atrial appendage plays a major role in arrhythmogenesis, thrombus formation, and associated stroke.
- Left atrial appendage plays an important role in homeostasis and hemodynamics via production of approximately 30% of atrial natriuretic peptide.
- Left atrial appendage occlusion leads to downregulation of the renin-angiontensin-aldosterone system which can lead to reduction in blood pressure due to increased natriuresis and diuresis.

INTRODUCTION

Atrial fibrillation (AF) is the most common cardiac arrhythmia in clinical practice and its incidence is increasing as the population ages.[1] AF is a leading cause of ischemic stroke.[2] Although oral anticoagulants (OACs) are effective in lowering the risk of stroke, approximately 10% of patients have an absolute or relative contraindication for anticoagulation. Complications such as intracranial bleeding and recurrent bleeding limit the use of warfarin and novel oral anticoagulants (NOACs) in others. As a result, almost half of the patients with AF at risk for stroke do not receive any anticoagulation.[3] Finally, among patients who do take anticoagulation for stroke prevention, approximately 50% discontinue the medication in 1 to 2 years.[4–6] Given that such a high percentage of patients with AF are at high risk of stroke and are not able to take anticoagulants, there is a large unmet need for alternative therapies in this area.

The left atrial appendage (LAA), a remnant of the primordial left atrium (LA), once considered to be merely an anatomic structure without clinical significance, has emerged as a key organ with distinct endocrinologic, mechanical, and physiologic properties.[7,8] LAA dysfunction plays a role in thrombus formation and is the most common source of thromboembolism in AF.[9] It serves as a reservoir during times of increased atrial pressure and volume and contributes to atrial compliance. In patients with AF, the LAA undergoes negative remodeling, which leads to a decrease in LAA compliance and decreased Doppler velocities, and makes it more prone to thrombus formation.

Financial Support: None.

[a] The Kansas City heart rhythm institution and research foundation, HCA MIDWEST HEALTH, Second Floor, 5100 W 110th St, Overland Park, KS 66211, USA; [b] Division of Cardiology, Department of Internal Medicine, MSC10-5550, 1 University of New Mexico, Albuquerque, NM 87131, USA; [c] Texas Cardiac Arrhythmia Institute, Center for Atrial Fibrillation at St. David's Medical Center, 1015 East 32nd Street, Suite 516, Austin, TX 78705, USA; [d] Department of Biomedical Engineering, University of Texas, 107 West Dean Keeton Street, Austin, TX 78712, USA

* Corresponding author.
E-mail address: dhanunjaya.lakkireddy@hcahealthcare.com

cardiacEP.theclinics.com

In addition, LAA plays a major role in homeostasis and hemodynamics: it produces approximately 30% of atrial natriuretic peptide (ANP), which causes natriuresis, and a decrease in blood pressure during times of increased LAA stretch. Furthermore, LAA serves as a site of nonpulmonary vein triggers in almost one-quarter of patients with persistent AF.[10]

Given its major role in arrhythmogenesis, thrombus formation, and associated stroke, the LAA has been a target of occlusion devices, both epicardial and endocardial. This review discusses the important role of LAA in systemic homeostasis and arrhythmogenesis; in addition, its potential role in blood pressure reduction is addressed.

ANATOMY OF THE LEFT ATRIAL APPENDAGE

The LAA originates from the primordial LA with variations in size and shape. In most patients the LAA extends between the anterior and lateral walls of the LA and its tip is directed anterosuperiorly, overlapping the left border of the right ventricular outflow tract or pulmonary trunk. The external appearance of the LAA is that of a flattened tubular structure with crenellations. The inner surface, by contrast, is lined by pectinate muscles that give it a trabecular appearance. There is a reduction in the number of LAA pectinate muscles in patients in sinus rhythm compared with those in AF. Four morphologic types have been documented: (1) cauliflower, (2) chicken wing, (3) cactus, and (4) wind sock.[11] The most common type is chicken wing. Cauliflower configuration is associated most with embolic events and has more complex internal characteristics such as extensive trabeculations, more irregular shape of the orifice, and short overall length.[12,13] Multiple lobes are common; almost half of the population has 2 lobes while 33% have 3 lobes.[10,14] In a study by Di Biase and colleagues,[15] the investigators revealed that extensive LAA trabeculations were associated with thromboembolic events. It was no surprise, then, that the vast majority of patients with the non–chicken-wing morphology had extensive trabeculations. Those with chicken-wing morphology have higher LAA flow velocities, which may explain the lower risk of thrombus formation in this morphology. This situation may assist in risk stratification of those patients with low CHA_2DS_2-VASc scores for whom decisions regarding anticoagulation have to be made.[16]

Previously the LAA was considered as a portion of the LA, but recently it has been shown to be a structure separate from the LA with distinct structural, physiologic, and hormonal properties.[13] In addition, the LAA is in close proximity to multiple critical structures such as the left circumflex artery, mitral valve, left superior pulmonary vein (PV), left superior vena cava, great cardiac vein, and ganglionic plexus. The safety of these structures comes into play when the LAA is excluded via endocardial or epicardial devices.[17,18] Furthermore, the fat pad around the LAA and the ganglionic plexi along the groove between the left superior PV and LAA plays a role in arrhythmogenesis. Speculation is that atrial remodeling during AF shifts the location of triggers from the PV to the LAA.[9]

HISTORICAL PERSPECTIVE

For many decades, the LAA has been implicated in the formation of thrombus and thromboembolic events.[19,20] In the 1950s, Belcher and Somerville[19,20] noted that LAA thrombus was present in greater than 60% of patients with a history of rheumatic valve disease undergoing mitral valvotomy who presented with thromboembolic events. LAA excision was first done during mitral valvotomy for this reason. Furthermore, Blackshear and Odell[21] found that the LAA was the source of thrombus in 90% of patients with nonvalvular AF. As the role of LAA in thrombogenesis evolved, interest in LAA exclusion gained popularity.

Interest in the physiologic and neurohormonal role of the LAA peaked following the Cox maze III procedure, which involved excision of the LAA. Patients became volume overloaded following the procedure because of a decrease in ANP secretion. This helped our understanding that LAA functions as a reservoir for ANP and acts as a major player in neurohormonal regulation.[22] The role of the LAA in neurohormonal regulation was further advanced by the HOMEOSTASIS study by Lakkireddy and colleagues[23] in which they studied the effects of LAA ligation on neurohormonal pathways. Lastly, given LAA and its role in thrombogenesis, mechanical devices for prophylactic closure of LAA for stroke prevention have gained popularity over the last 2 decades.

LEFT ATRIAL APPENDAGE REMODELING AND THROMBUS FORMATION

Significant LAA remodeling occurs in AF patients and contributes to the initiation and maintenance of AF. While the chicken-wing LAA morphology is most common, in one study of patients with persistent AF, significant remodeling led the morphology to change to non–chicken-wing type.[24] MRI is a useful tool to assess cardiac remodeling, and late gadolinium enhancement (LGE), in particular, can be used to assess fibrosis. It is interesting that in areas of the LAA with the highest LGE, there was increased arrhythmia recurrence and up to 4-fold more in patients in the highest LGE group. Furthermore, over a 5-year follow-up, patients with advanced atrial fibrosis had a higher AF ablation procedural failure rate.[25]

This is a key finding and underscores the importance of LAA remodeling that takes place. On the contrary, LAA exclusion via the LARIAT procedure has shown reverse LA remodeling and improved LA mechanical function.[26]

The LAA is prone to thrombus formation, with approximately 91% to 100% of thrombi in non-valvular AF formed in the LAA.[15] Several factors contribute to thrombus formation. A decrease in left ventricular contractility such as occurs in heart failure leads to reduced and stagnant flow, which then leads to thrombus formation. Patients with chronic AF have larger LAA volumes and greater endocardial thickening with fibrous tissue compared with those without AF. These findings may play a role in thrombus formation in chronic AF.[27] In addition, in AF a prothrombotic state ensues marked by activation of interleukin-6, platelet aggregation, thrombin complexes, and d-dimer.[28,29] Furthermore, reduced LAA contractility and function in AF lead to dilation of the LAA, stagnation of flow, and increased risk of thrombosis.[12] LAA morphology also plays a role in thrombosis; Yamamoto and colleagues[30] reported that the number of LAA lobes correlates with a complex LAA morphology and is a significant risk factor for LAA thrombus.

ROLE OF LEFT ATRIAL APPENDAGE IN SYSTEMIC HOMEOSTASIS

The LAA is a dynamic structure that contributes both passively and actively to the LA during the cardiac cycle. As the left ventricle dilates during diastole, the intrapericardial space is filled, which causes LAA emptying by compressing the inferomedial wall of the LAA. In addition, ventricular filling creates a suction effect, which causes emptying of the LA and LAA. The LAA serves as a reservoir during ventricular systole, a channel for blood flow transitioning from the PVs to the LA.[31] Whether it functions as an active or passive muscle was questioned, although recent evidence suggests that it is an active muscle because it has prominent ridges and surgeons have reported active contraction during the time of surgery.[32,33]

ATRIAL NATRIURETIC PEPTIDE–RELATED EFFECTS

The LAA produces both ANP and brain natriuretic peptide (BNP) in response to stretch in the LA and LAA. Approximately 30% of ANP and a smaller amount of BNP is secreted from LAA. They are in turn involved in systemic homeostasis by promoting natriuresis, diuresis, and vasodilation. Volume overload leads to distention of the LAA, which leads to secretion of ANP and excretion of potassium and chloride at the level of the kidneys. ANP inhibits renin, leading to decreased angiotensin II (ATII), decreased aldosterone, and subsequent diuresis and natriuresis. Vasodilation mediated by lack of ATII leads to a drop in systemic blood pressure[34–37] (**Fig. 1**).

Of interest is that both atrial appendages respond to stretch receptors; hence, removal of both the appendages has a greater impact on ANP secretion than the removal of one appendage.[12] These physiologic effects were observed during the Cox maze III procedure, which involved excision of the LAA along with the tip of the right atrial appendage (RAA). Patients went into heart failure immediately afterward owing to the significant decrease in ANP levels. Because of this complication, it was noted that perhaps leaving the RAA intact would ameliorate the observed fluid overload. Hence, removal of the LAA without removing the RAA was advocated because the RAA would still produce some amount of ANP.[22]

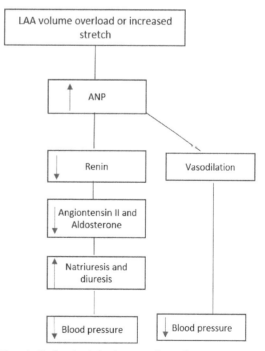

Fig. 1. Pathophysiologic sequelae of LAA volume overload or increased stretch. ANP, atrial natriuretic peptide; LAA, left atrial appendage.

DOWNREGULATION OF THE RENIN-ANGIOTENSIN-ALDOSTERONE SYSTEM

Occlusion of the appendage has multiple downstream physiologic effects. Wozakowska-Kapłon and Opolski[38] showed that plasma ANP decreased after successful cardioversion of persistent AF. This was corroborated by studies of Dixen and colleagues[39] and Fujiwara and colleagues,[40] both of which showed an association between AF and elevated natriuretic peptides. These findings were also observed in patients who underwent epicardial LAA occlusion.[23] In addition, the LAA HOMEOSTASIS study by Lakkireddy and colleagues[23] showed that adrenaline and noradrenaline levels decreased in patients undergoing LAA epicardial closure. However, there was no change in their levels following endocardial occlusion. This can be explained by the decreased sympathetic drive that ensues after LAA closure and the downstream physiologic effects.[23] Of importance in this study is that ANP and BNP levels increased back to baseline after 3 months in the epicardial occlusion group. However, the renin-angiotensin-aldosterone system (RAAS) continued to be downregulated, perhaps because of the autonomic circuits that were affected from the LAA fat pad necrosis after epicardial occlusion (**Table 1**). This highlights an important concept, namely that there may be another physiologic process besides ANP that is affecting RAAS. One hypothesis for downregulation of RAAS after appendage ligation could be a decrease in angiotensin-converting enzyme and ATII type 1

receptors in the LA, which are upregulated in patients with AF.[41] An interesting concept is that upregulation of the RAAS, as seen with AF, causes atrial fibrosis and myocyte hypertrophy over time. Downregulation of RAAS, as observed in LAA occlusion, can serve to induce positive remodeling and improve hemodynamics.[42–45] **Fig. 2** illustrates the impact of LAA exclusion.

LEFT ATRIAL APPENDAGE AND ITS ROLE IN ARRHYTHMOGENESIS

PVs play a major role in the initiation and maintenance of AF, especially in paroxysmal AF. Persistent AF has varying success rates (46%–59%) with PV isolation alone, as seen in the STAR AFII trial suggesting non-PV triggers for AF.[46,47] It was not until 2010 that LAA was found to be a major contributor to AF in this population. The LAA of patients with AF who underwent surgical ablation and LAA amputation showed that LAA was characterized by thick interstitial fibrotic bands and changes in conduction velocity, which served to form an arrhythmogenic substrate for re-entry.[48] Di Biase and colleagues[49] in their study in 2010 looked at 987 patients who underwent repeat catheter ablation for AF and showed that 27% of patients had firing from the LAA and that in 8.7% of patients the LAA was the only source of AF. In 2011 Hocini and colleagues[50] reaffirmed these findings, confirming that LAA was a source of ectopic triggers and re-entrant atrial tachycardia in patients with persistent AF. Another interesting fact is that LAA can be a source of arrhythmia in

Table 1
Impact of closure of left atrial appendage on the adrenergic system and renin-angiotensin-aldosterone system

Epicardial Device	Preprocedure	3 Months Post Procedure	P Value
Adrenaline (pg/mL)	60.49	31.80	<.01
Noradrenaline (ng/mL)	73.85	36.40	<.01
Aldosterone (ng/dL)	4.22	0.72	<.01
Renin (pg/mL)	52.90	18.30	<.01
Endocardial Device	**Preprocedure**	**3 Months Post Procedure**	**P Value**
Adrenaline (pg/mL)	14.50	13.82	.09
Noradrenaline (ng/dL)	50.36	38.43	.68
Aldosterone (ng/dL)	13.34	13.63	.40
Renin (pg/mL)	22.04	25.42	.19

Adapted from Lakkireddy D, Turagam M, Afzal MR, et al. Left Atrial Appendage Closure and Systemic Homeostasis: The LAA HOMEOSTASIS Study. J Am Coll Cardiol. 2018 Jan 16;71(2):135-144; with permission.

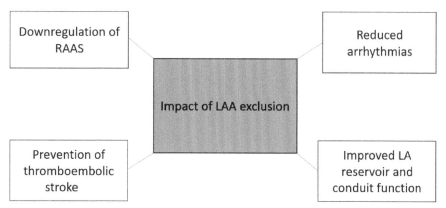

Fig. 2. Impact of LAA exclusion. LA, left atrium; LAA, left atrial appendage; RAAS, renin-angiotensin-aldosterone system. (*Adapted from* Turagam, MK, Velagapudi P, Kar S et al. Cardiovascular Therapies Targeting Left Atrial Appendage. Journal of the American College of Cardiology, 72(4), 448–463; with permission.)

approximately 3% of young patients without heart disease.[51-53]

In the study by Starck and colleagues[54] in which 10 patients underwent epicardial LAA occlusion, results showed complete electrical isolation of the LAA in all cases. Results of the BELIEF Trial in 2015 showed that patients with long-standing persistent AF who underwent empiric LAA isolation along with extensive ablation had improved long-term freedom from arrhythmia recurrence.[10] In addition, a meta-analysis by AlTurki and colleagues[55] showed that LAA isolation added to PV isolation reduced AF recurrence. Yorgun and colleagues[56] studied 100 patients with persistent AF and found that LAA isolation as an adjunct to PV isolation improved 1-year outcomes. Lastly, a large meta-analysis by Friedman and colleagues[57] in 2018 showed that LAA electrical isolation was associated with a significant reduction in recurrent atrial tachycardia and AF. This is in part because atrial remodeling over time shifts the location of the AF triggers from the PV to other areas, likely the LAA. Moreover, the LAA is innervated by autonomic ganglia, which play a crucial role in arrhythmogenesis and can be affected by LAA ligation.[58]

LAA occlusion plays a role in managing longstanding persistent AF. LAA ligation using LARIAT causes infarct of the LAA resulting from obstruction of epicardial blood flow. This leads to transmural necrosis and decreased voltage, thereby decreasing the available substrate for AF.[9,59] Endocardial occlusion with the Watchman device, on the other hand, does not lead to necrosis of the LAA. Hence, there is no effect on AF substrate.[9] Residual leaks or communication between the LA and LAA are a known complication of percutaneous LAA closure. The incidence of leaks after a LARIAT procedure ranges from 0% to 24%. Leaks after epicardial ligation can potentially reduce the

long-term efficacy of this procedure and can have arrhythmogenic implications.[60] In a study by Turagam and colleagues,[61] the investigators observed that small leaks (1–3 mm) were associated with no LAA electrical activity and the results were comparable with those from patients who had complete LAA ligation without any residual leak. Larger leaks (4–5 mm), by contrast, demonstrated residual electrical activity during catheter ablation. Interestingly, recurrence of AF was similar between the 2 groups in this study, although the sample size was small and the result not statistically significant. Incomplete ischemic remodeling probably occurs in large leaks, which leads to a lower reduction in LAA size and volume and thus to persistence in electrical activity. On the contrary, smaller leaks lead to a greater reduction in LAA size and volume as well as reduction in the active muscle fiber, which then causes a reduction in the electrical activity.[61-63]

LEFT ATRIAL APPENDAGE AND BEYOND

Given the downregulation of the RAAS leading to increased insulin levels that is seen with LAA ligation, there may be potential benefit in patients with AF who have type 2 diabetes. Downregulation of the RAAS also leads to a decrease in blood pressure owing to natriuresis and diuresis.[23] However, this was only seen in patients who underwent epicardial LAA occlusion. In the LAA HOMEOSTASIS study by Lakkireddy and colleagues,[23] a decrease in adrenaline, noradrenaline, renin, and aldosterone was noted at 3 months in the epicardial occlusion group whereas similar changes were not observed in the endocardial group. These findings were confirmed with Turagam and colleagues,[42] who reported a reduction in systolic and diastolic blood pressure at 3 months and

1 year in patients who underwent epicardial LAA exclusion. Similar reductions in blood pressure have not been seen with endocardial devices, likely because there is a lack of LAA necrosis, the blood supply to the LAA is intact, and the RAAS is not downregulated. In addition, Ramirez and colleagues[64] examined the effects of systolic blood pressure in patients with AF who underwent catheter ablation and found that successful catheter ablation led to a decrease in systolic blood pressure.

CONFLICT OF INTEREST

None.

REFERENCES

1. Morillo CA, Banerjee A, Perel P, et al. Atrial fibrillation: the current epidemic. J Geriatr Cardiol 2017; 14(3):195–203.
2. Bunch TJ, May HT, Bair TL, et al. Atrial fibrillation ablation patients have long-term stroke rates similar to patients without atrial fibrillation regardless of CHADS2 score. Heart Rhythm 2013;10:1272–7.
3. Panaich S, Holmes DR. Left atrial appendage occlusion. 2017. American College of Cardiology Expert Analysis. Available at: http://www.acc.org/latest-in-cardiology/articles/2017/01/31/13/08/left-atrial-appendage-occlusion.
4. Connolly SJ, Ezekowitz MD, Yusuf S, et al. Dabigatran versus warfarin in patients with atrial fibrillation. N Engl J Med 2009;361:1139–51.
5. Granger CB, Alexander JH, McMurray JJ, et al. Apixaban versus warfarin in patients with atrial fibrillation. N Engl J Med 2011;365:981–92.
6. Jazayeri MA, Vuddanda V, Parikh V, et al. Five years of keeping a watch on the left atrial appendage-how has the WATCHMAN fared? J Thorac Dis 2016; 8(12):E1726–33.
7. Turagam MK, Velagapudi P, Kar S, et al. Cardiovascular therapies targeting left atrial appendage. J Am Coll Cardiol 2018;72(4):448–63.
8. Delgado V, Di Biase L, Leung M, et al. Structure and function of the left atrium and left atrial appendage: AF and stroke implications. J Am Coll Cardiol 2017; 70(25):3157–72.
9. Lakkireddy D, Mahankali AS, Kanmanthareddy A, et al. Left atrial appendage ligation and ablation for persistent atrial fibrillation. The LAALA-AF registry. JACC Clin Electrophysiol 2015;1(3):153–60.
10. Di Biase L, Burkhardt JD, Mohanty P, et al. Left atrial appendage isolation in patients with longstanding persistent AF undergoing catheter ablation: BELIEF trial. J Am Coll Cardiol 2016;68(18):1929–40.
11. Lupercio F, Carlos Ruiz J, Briceno DF, et al. Left atrial appendage morphology assessment for risk stratification of embolic stroke in patients with atrial fibrillation: a meta-analysis. Heart Rhythm 2016; 13(7):1402–9.
12. Beigel R, Wunderlich NC, Ho SY, et al. The left atrial appendage: anatomy, function, and noninvasive evaluation. JACC Cardiovasc Imaging 2014;7(12): 1251–65.
13. Saygi S. Atrial fibrillation and the role of LAA in pathophysiology and clinical outcomes? J Atr Fibrillation 2012;5(3):480.
14. Veinot JP, Harrity PJ, Gentile F, et al. Anatomy of the normal left atrial appendage: a quantitative study of age-related changes in 500 autopsy hearts: implications for echocardiographic examination. Circulation 1997;96:3112–5.
15. Di Biase L, Natale A, Romero J. Thrombogenic and arrhythmogenic roles of the left atrial appendage in atrial fibrillation. Circulation 2018;138(18):2036–50.
16. Fukushima K, Fukushima N, Kato K, et al. Correlation between left atrial appendage morphology and flow velocity in patients with paroxysmal atrial fibrillation. Eur Heart J Cardiovasc Imaging 2016;17(1):59–66.
17. Evora PRB, Menardi AC, Celotto AC, et al. The left atrial appendage revised. Braz J Cardiovasc Surg 2017;32(6):517–22.
18. DeSimone CV, Prakriti BG, Tri J, et al. A review of the relevant embryology, pathohistology, and anatomy of the left atrial appendage for the invasive cardiac electrophysiologist. J Atr Fibrillation 2015;8(2):1129.
19. Chatterjee S, Alexander JC, Pearson PJ, et al. Left atrial appendage occlusion: lessons learned from surgical and transcatheter experiences. Ann Thorac Surg 2011;92:2283–92.
20. Belcher JR, Somerville W. Systemic embolism and left auricular thrombosis in relation to mitral valvotomy. Br Med J 1955;2:1000–3.
21. Blackshear JL, Odell JA. Appendage obliteration to reduce stroke in cardiac surgical patients with atrial fibrillation. Ann Thorac Surg 1996;61:755–9.
22. Hanke T. Surgical management of the left atrial appendage: a must or a myth? Eur J Cardiothorac Surg 2018;53(suppl_1):i33–8.
23. Lakkireddy D, Turagam M, Afzal MR, et al. Left atrial appendage closure and systemic homeostasis: the LAA HOMEOSTASIS study. J Am Coll Cardiol 2018;71(2):135–44.
24. Kishima H, Mine T, Takahashi S, et al. Morphologic remodeling of left atrial appendage in patients with atrial fibrillation. Heart Rhythm 2016; 13(9):1823–8.
25. Suksaranjit P, Marrouche NF, Han FT, et al. Relation of left atrial appendage remodeling by magnetic resonance imaging and outcome of ablation for atrial fibrillation. Am J Cardiol 2018;122(1):83–8.
26. Dar T, Afzal MR, Yarlagadda B, et al. Mechanical function of the left atrium is improved with epicardial ligation of the left atrial appendage: insights from the

LAFIT-LARIAT registry. Heart Rhythm 2018;15(7): 955–9.

27. Shirani J, Alaeddini J. Structural remodeling of the left atrial appendage in patients with chronic non-valvular atrial fibrillation: implications for thrombus formation, systemic embolism, and assessment by transesophageal echocardiography. Cardiovasc Pathol 2000;9(2):95–101.

28. Khan AA, Lip GYH. The prothrombotic state in atrial fibrillation: pathophysiological and management implications. Cardiovasc Res 2019;115(1):31–45.

29. Conway DS, Buggins P, Hughes E, et al. Relationship of interleukin-6 and C-reactive protein to the prothrombotic state in chronic atrial fibrillation. J Am Coll Cardiol 2004;43:2075–82.

30. Yamamoto M, Seo Y, Kawamatsu N, et al. Complex left atrial appendage morphology and left atrial appendage thrombus formation in patients with atrial fibrillation. Circ Cardiovasc Imaging 2014;7: 337–43.

31. Mehrzad R, Rajab M, Spodick DH. The three integrated phases of left atrial macrophysiology and their interactions. Int J Mol Sci 2014;15(9):15146–60.

32. Regazzoli D, Ancona F, Trevisi N, et al. Left atrial appendage: physiology, pathology, and role as a therapeutic target. Biomed Res Int 2015;2015:13.

33. Al-Saady NM, Abel OA, Camm AJ. Left atrial appendage: structure, function, and role in thromboembolism. Heart 1999;82:547–55.

34. Wilber DJ. Neurohormonal regulation and the left atrial appendage. J Am Coll Cardiol 2018;71(2): 145–7.

35. Potter RL, Abbey-Hosch S, Dickey DM. Natriuretic peptides, their receptors, and cyclic guanosine monophosphate-dependent signaling functions. Endocr Rev 2006;27:47–72.

36. Saito Y. Roles of atrial natriuretic peptide and its therapeutic use. J Cardiol 2010;56:262–70.

37. Song W, Wang H, Wu Q. Atrial natriuretic peptide in cardiovascular biology and disease (NPPA). Gene 2015;569:1–6.

38. Wozakowska-Kapłon B, Opolski G. Concomitant recovery of atrial mechanical and endocrine function after cardioversion in patients with persistent atrial fibrillation. J Am Coll Cardiol 2003;41(10):1716–20.

39. Dixen U, Ravn L, Soeby-Rasmussen C, et al. Raised plasma aldosterone and natriuretic peptides in atrial fibrillation. Cardiology 2006;108(1):35–9.

40. Fujiwara H, Ishikura M, Nagata S, et al. Plasma atrial natriuretic peptide response to direct current cardioversion of atrial fibrillation in patients with mitral stenosis. J Am Coll Cardiol 1993;22(2):575–80.

41. Iravanian S, Dudley SC Jr. The renin-angiotensin-aldosterone system (RAAS) and cardiac arrhythmias. Heart Rhythm 2008;5(6 Suppl):S12–7 [published correction appears in Heart Rhythm 2008; 5(10):1499].

42. Turagam MK, Vuddanda V, Verberkmoes N, et al. Epicardial left atrial appendage exclusion reduces blood pressure in patients with atrial fibrillation and hypertension. J Am Coll Cardiol 2018;72(12): 1346–53.

43. Reil JC, Hohl M, Selejan S, et al. Aldosterone promotes atrial fibrillation. Eur Heart J 2012;33: 2098–108.

44. Pathak R. Structural and functional remodeling of the left atrium: clinical and therapeutic implications for atrial fibrillation. J Atr Fibrillation 2013;6(4):986.

45. Yongjun Q, Huanzhang S, Wenxia Z, et al. From changes in local RAAS to structural remodeling of the left atrium: a beautiful cycle in atrial fibrillation. Herz 2015;40(3):514–20.

46. Verma A, Jiang CY, Betts TR, et al. Approaches to catheter ablation for persistent atrial fibrillation. N Engl J Med 2015;372:1812–22.

47. Kirchhof P, Calkins H. Catheter ablation in patients with persistent atrial fibrillation. Eur Heart J 2017; 38(1):20–6.

48. Nishimura M, Lupercio-Lopez F, Hsu JC. Left atrial appendage electrical isolation as a target in atrial fibrillation. JACC Clin Electrophysiol 2019;5(4): 407–16.

49. Di Base L, Burkhardt JD, Mohanty P, et al. Left atrial appendage: an underrecognized trigger site of atrial fibrillation. Circulation 2010;122(2):109–18.

50. Hocini M, Shah AJ, Nault I, et al. Localized reentry within the left atrial appendage: arrhythmogenic role in patients undergoing ablation of persistent atrial fibrillation. Heart Rhythm 2011;8(12): 1853–61.

51. Naksuk N, Padmanabhan D, Yogeswaran V, et al. Left atrial appendage: embryology, anatomy, physiology, arrhythmia and therapeutic intervention. JACC Clin Electrophysiol 2016;2(4):403–12.

52. Wang YL, Li XB, Quan X, et al. Focal atrial tachycardia originating from the left atrial appendage: electrocardiographic and electrophysiologic characterization and long-term outcomes of radiofrequency ablation. J Cardiovasc Electrophysiol 2007; 18:459–64, 37.

53. Yamada T, Murakami Y, Yoshida Y, et al. Electrophysiologic and electrocardiographic characteristics and radiofrequency catheter ablation of focal atrial tachycardia originating from the left atrial appendage. Heart Rhythm 2007;4:1284–91.

54. Starck CT, Steffel J, Emmert MY, et al. Epicardial left atrial appendage clip occlusion also provides the electrical isolation of the left atrial appendage. Interact Cardiovasc Thorac Surg 2012;15(3):416–8.

55. AlTurki A, Huynh T, Dawas A, et al. Left atrial appendage isolation in atrial fibrillation catheter ablation: a meta-analysis. J Arrhythm 2018;34(5):478–84.

56. Yorgun H, Canpolat U, Kocyigit D, et al. Left atrial appendage isolation in addition to pulmonary vein

isolation in persistent atrial fibrillation: one-year clinical outcome after cryoballoon-based ablation. Europace 2017;19(5):758–68.

57. Friedman DJ, Black-Maier EW, Barnett AS, et al. Left atrial appendage electrical isolation for treatment of recurrent atrial fibrillation: a meta-analysis. JACC Clin Electrophysiol 2018;4(1):112–20.

58. Linz D, Ukena C, Mahfoud F, et al. Atrial autonomic innervation. J Am Coll Cardiol 2014;63(3): 215–24.

59. Han FT, Bartus K, Lakkireddy D, et al. The effects of LAA ligation on LAA electrical activity. Heart Rhythm 2014;11:864–70.

60. Yarlagadda B, Parikh V, Dar T, et al. Leaks after left atrial appendage ligation with Lariat device: incidence, pathophysiology, clinical implications and methods of closure—a case based discussion. J Atr Fibrillation 2017;10(3):1725.

61. Turagam M, Atkins D, Earnest M, et al. Anatomical and electrical remodeling with incomplete left atrial appendage ligation: results from the LAALA-AF registry. J Cardiovasc Electrophysiol 2017;28(12): 1433–42.

62. Kreidieh B, Rojas F, Schurmann P, et al. Left atrial appendage remodeling after Lariat left atrial appendage ligation. Circ Arrhythm Electrophysiol 2015;8(6):1351–8.

63. Gianni C, Biase LD, Trivedi C, et al. Clinical implications of leaks following left atrial appendage ligation with the LARIAT device. JACC Cardiovasc Interv 2016;9(10):1051–7.

64. Ramirez A, Pacchia CF, Sanders NA, et al. The effects of radio-frequency ablation on blood pressure control in patients with atrial fibrillation and hypertension. J Interv Card Electrophysiol 2012;35(3): 285–91.

When to Refer Patients for Left Atrial Appendage Closure

Christopher R. Ellis, MD, FHRS[a],*, Gregory G. Jackson, MD[b]

KEYWORDS

- Atrial fibrillation • Left atrial appendage (LAA) • Hemorrhagic stroke • Anticoagulation • HAS-BLED
- Major bleeding • Nonvalvular atrial fibrillation

KEY POINTS

- LAA occlusion devices are becoming increasingly considered an alternative to oral anticoagulation for patients with nonvalvular atrial fibrillation and high bleeding risk.
- Selection of appropriate candidates for an LAAC device are based on both previous bleeding events, perceived future bleeding risk, compliance with anticoagulation, and concomitant disease therapy (ie, surgical LAA occlusion).
- Little is known about safety and efficacy of LAAC devices in patients with bioprosthetic tissue aortic or mitral valve replacement.
- A truly OAC/DOAC contraindicated patient can still be considered for LAAC with appropriate device selection and antiplatelet therapy alone after implant (ASAP registry, ASAP-TOO trial, Amulet IDE trial, surgical or epicardial LAA closure).

INTRODUCTION

Atrial fibrillation (AF) is the most common cardiac arrhythmia in the United States with an estimated 5 million patients affected. As part of the management of such patients, stroke prevention is an important consideration for each provider to address. Based on risk stratification scores, CHADS2 and CHA2DS2VASc being the most common, clinicians can be guided to know which patients are at higher risk of stroke and require stroke prophylaxis with oral anticoagulation (OAC). Specifically, the current recommendation is that patients with CHADS2 and CHA2DS2VASc ≥ 2 should receive stroke prophylaxis.[1,2] Warfarin was the mainstay of OAC for stroke prophylaxis until the last several years during which direct OACs (DOACs) have become a mainstay. This shift relates the issues of consideration warfarin therapy and the results of multiple large randomized trials including RE-LY in 2009, ROCKET AF in 2011, and ENGAGE AF-TIMI 48 and ARISTOTLE in 2011, all of which documented excellent outcomes for using dabigatran, rivaroxaban, edoxaban, and apixaban, respectively, for nonvalvular atrial fibrillation (NVAF).[3–6]

Based on the criteria for CHADS2 score, approximately 3 million US patients would be candidates for oral anticoagulation with either warfarin or a DOAC. Data from the PINNACLE registry confirm that about 50% of CHADS2Vasc greater than 2 patients with AF are actually taking or prescribed oral anticoagulation, identifying a very large at-risk population of candidates for potential left atrial appendage closure (LAAC).[7] In addition, many patients are unable to tolerate lifelong

[a] LAA Closure Program, Vanderbilt Heart and Vascular Institute, Vanderbilt University Medical Center, Medical Center East- 5414 (Suite 5209), 1211 21st Avenue South, Nashville, TN 37232-8802, USA; [b] Internal Medicine Residency Program, Vanderbilt University Medical Center, 1211 21st Avenue South, Nashville, TN 37232-8802, USA
* Corresponding author.
E-mail addresses: Christopher.ellis@vumc.org; cellisvandyep@gmail.com

Card Electrophysiol Clin 12 (2020) 29–37
https://doi.org/10.1016/j.ccep.2019.11.005
1877-9182/20/© 2019 Elsevier Inc. All rights reserved.

anticoagulation because of previous medical conditions, bleeding risk, or other intolerances to anticoagulation. Finally, long-term compliance with anticoagulant therapy for stroke prevention in this setting is at best 60%. Because most strokes (>90%) associated with AF are presumed to originate from an embryologic remnant of the left atrium, the left atrial appendage (LAA), ligation or occlusion of the LAA was devised to eliminate clot formation, and possible migration that could result in AF-related embolic stroke.[8] Percutaneous LAA device-based closure as an option for stroke prevention for NVAF with the Watchman LAAC device (Boston Scientific Inc, Natick, MA), gained approval by the Food and Drug Administration (FDA) in 2015 as an alternative to oral anticoagulation following the PROTECT AF (2009) and PREVAIL (2014) studies.[9,10]

Novel procedures and therapies involving LAAC on the horizon may yet broaden the scope of treatment with LAAC. However, the decision of when to refer a patient for LAAC may not be clear for many providers. The purpose of this article is to aid the clinician in understanding current guidelines for LAAC, patient-specific criteria that need to be met to qualify for LAAC, and how the post-implant drug regimen affects these decisions.

CURRENT GUIDELINES AS OUTLINED BY CENTERS FOR MEDICARE AND MEDICAID, US FOOD AND DRUG ADMINISTRATION, AND AMERICAN COLLEGE OF CARDIOLOGY/ AMERICAN HEART ASSOCIATION FOR LEFT ATRIAL APPENDAGE CLOSURE

Prevention of stroke is the driving force for consideration of OAC or DOAC versus LAAC but needs to be weighed against the possible adverse outcomes related to anticoagulation. The most significant adverse event, and most commonly encountered by the clinician, is bleeding. Validated scoring systems, such as the HAS-BLED score is commonly used, and patients who qualify for LAAC typically have a score of ≥3, portending a 3.74% yearly risk of a major bleed while on warfarin.[11] Prospective registries of adherence to DOAC therapy, and several large randomized clinical trial trials support a risk profile of 2% to 3% per annum major bleed risk in all comers with a less than 1% risk for intracranial hemorrhage. Over time, even in clinical trials, there is about a 40% drop off in compliance with therapy per year.[3,4,6]

When the Watchman device was first approved in 2015, the Centers for Medicare and Medicaid (CMS) issued a memorandum detailing which patients would be approved for left atrial appendage closure. The criteria include (1) CHA2DS2VASc score ≥2 for men and CHA2DS2-VASc score ≥3 for women and (2) formal "shared decision-making" and determination that the patient is "suitable for short-term warfarin, but deemed unable to take long-term oral anticoagulation." In addition, it requires that the procedure be performed by an interventionalist who has performed ≥25 occlusion procedures over a 2-year period.[11] Alternatively, the FDA states that the Watchman device is indicated in patients who are deemed to be suitable for warfarin but in whom there is "appropriate rationale to seek a non-pharmacologic alternative to warfarin."[12] A specific criteria for what patient or condition is an appropriate rationale is vague, and the focus of this review. Oddly, an objective bleeding risk calculation is not a part of LAAC coverage, thus it may be appropriate in some cases to refer a patient with a HAS-BLED score of 1 or 2 for closure.

American College of Cardiology/American Heart Association (ACC/AHA) guidelines updated and released in 2019 dictate that the standard of care is still that those who qualify for anticoagulation should be treated with warfarin or DOAC, where eligible, for stroke prophylaxis.[13] The guidelines do recognize that treatment with an OAC is not plausible for many patients and that LAAC could be a viable option for such patients. However, the best recommendation category remains a class IIb, based on limited randomized controlled trial data with competing therapies. Thus, the somewhat nonspecific criteria outlined by the CMS, FDA, and ACC/AHA provide little help to identify which patients actually should be evaluated for LAAC. Clinical factors supportive of considering LAAC in specific clinical scenarios are discussed in detail below.

ADDITIONAL CONSIDERATION ON COMPETING STROKE RISK

The risk of AF embolic stroke needs to be significant enough for the risk of the LAAC procedure, or the presence of the device, not to outweigh the overall clinical benefit. Typically the HAS-BLED score will increase in parallel with the CHADS2Vasc score, and that alone may identify an appropriate patient base for LAAC consideration (high CHADS2Vasc >3, HAS-BLED >3). For example, a female patient older than 65 years, with hypertension (uncontrolled >160 mm), and having had a previous stroke would have a CHADS2Vasc of 5 and HAS-BLED of 3. The provider must also consider the effect of a 2% procedural risk (vascular injury, pericardial effusion, stroke, and device embolization) plus a 1-year 3% to 4% risk of device-related thrombus (DRT) associated with the Watchman device. The accompanying 4- to 5-fold odds ratio for embolic ischemic events with DRT could mitigate the stroke prevention benefit of Watchman for some patients,[14,15] although most patients with DRT do not develop an ischemic event, and DRT itself can usually be treated with a short trial of anticoagulation with resolution.

Known associated factors increasing the risk for DRT include depressed ejection fraction with systolic heart failure, persistent AF, large LAA volume before LAAC, and likely inherent prothrombotic states, which are poorly studied in this population. Patients with persistent AF referred for an endocardial LAAC device with complex LAA anatomy, dense spontaneous echo contrast or sludge, and a depressed left ventricular ejection fraction (LVEF) should certainly be "able to tolerate" short-term anticoagulation after the device is implanted.[15] Otherwise the patient may be subjected to a high-risk scenario, such as recent conversion from AF to sinus and a fresh LAAC device followed by a major bleed, cessation of anticoagulation, and then development of a DRT with a potential for a large embolic stroke.

Apart from hypercoagulable states, patients with a heavy burden of atherosclerotic plaque in the ascending aorta, carotid or vertebral arteries, a patent foramen ovale (PFO) with right to left shunt, and patients with left ventricular thrombus would seem unlikely to benefit greatly from the Watchman LAAC device. However, a recent analysis of high CHADS2Vasc subjects (5 or higher) undergoing LAAC at the Cleveland Clinic supports that the benefits of Watchman remain, and in fact, may be enhanced for high-risk Watchman recipients compared with estimated stroke and bleed risk based on CHADS2Vasc historical data.[16] A clinical scenario that is beyond the scope of typical indications for LAAC may include the patient at high risk for AF stroke in whom a decision could be made to occlude the LAA for solely for added stroke prevention. Patients with a known cardioembolic stroke while on anticoagulation, or those with a high-risk LAA (low LAA ejection velocity, heavy spontaneous echo contrast, "sludge," or known LAA thrombus) could possibly have added benefit from LAAC, all while remaining on systemic oral anticoagulation, presuming they tolerate it.

INDICATIONS FOR CONSIDERATION OF LEFT ATRIAL APPENDAGE CLOSURE
Nonvalvular Atrial Fibrillation

Updated guidelines in 2019 by the ACC/AHA-defined valvular heart disease as it relates to AF as patients having either moderate to severe mitral stenosis, or patients who have undergone artificial heart valve replacement (prosthetic or mechanical valves). This distinction is important in the consideration of patients being managed for AF. First, in patients with valvular heart disease, anticoagulation with warfarin is the current standard of practice. The off-label use of DOACs for patients with bioprosthetic valves is increasing steadily but these patients were excluded from large randomized clinical trials. Patients with mechanical valves continue to require dose-adjusted warfarin after failure of the RE-ALIGN study.[17] Likewise, as indicated by the FDA labeling, only patients with NVAF are considered for LAAC with the Watchman device, thus excluding those with moderate to severe mitral disease or those with artificial mechanical valves. Similar to the use of DOACs, indications for LAAC in patients with bioprosthetic valves or those with significant mitral valve disease warrants formal study.

Increased Stroke Risk

Patients with NVAF who are at low risk for stroke (CHA2DS2-VASc <2) would be deferred LAAC as an option, and treatment would typically entail single antiplatelet therapy (ie, aspirin) or no therapy. It is interesting to note that although LAAC was approved by CMS as an alternative for stroke prophylaxis in the setting of anticoagulant failure or intolerance, the initial studies evaluating Watchman did not require a bleeding event for inclusion. Initially the PROTECT AF trial randomized 707 patients with NVAF and CHADS2 score $\geq$1 to LAAC with the Watchman device versus warfarin in a ratio of 2:1.[10] The risk of hemorrhagic stroke was much less after LAAC (1/708.4 versus 6/373.4, relative risk [RR] = 0.09; 95% CI, 0.00–0.45) and there seemed to be a trend toward decreased all-cause mortality as a result of this in the Watchman group (1/708.4 versus 18/374.9, RR = 0.62; 95% CI, 0.34–1.24). Adverse events were more common in the procedural group leading to initial delays in FDA approval (6 air embolic events included as early ischemic strokes). Therefore, although approved for OAC failure, there may be a role for LAAC at the initial onset of AF before any anticoagulation when the perceived risk-benefit ratio favors LAAC, particularly a patient with a previous intracranial hemorrhage but new onset AF. In these patients the clinical and patient decision may be to proceed to LAAC as the initial therapy.

Relative Contraindication to Oral Anticoagulation

The most common indication for consideration of LAAC is intolerance to OAC. As described above, at present all patients considered for Watchman must demonstrate some inability to take OAC long term. There are a variety of scenarios where a patient may be deemed unsuitable for OAC, some of the most common are outlined below (**Table 1**).

All of the clinical scenarios in **Table 1** would meet the criteria under the CMS guidelines for inability to tolerate long-term anticoagulation when paired with a shared decision-making process via a nonimplanting physician. It is important to mention that CMS guidelines indicate that patient's being evaluated for LAAC must be "suitable for short-term warfarin." This stems from the current clinical practice of treating a patient with 3 to 6 weeks of oral anticoagulation (typically warfarin) before placement of the Watchman device. This strategy was identified to enhance the potential for endothelialization of the device after implantation. After the device is placed, the patient would continue on OAC for 45 days, at which point they would undergo transesophageal echocardiography (TEE) for visualization of the device and LAA. If at that time there is a less than 5-mm leak surrounding the device and no DRT, OAC could be safely discontinued. Dual antiplatelet therapy for 6 months is then followed by aspirin only indefinitely. A significant shift to the use of DOACs post-LAAC has been supported by observational data, and new clinical trial protocols (**Table 2**) have changed to improve the post-implant drug regimen.[18,19] We typically would still consider LAAC referral in a high-risk AF patient who has never taken warfarin, or is not willing to take short-term warfarin.

Table 1	
Relative contraindications for anticoagulation (indications for left atrial appendage closure referral)	
System	**Relative Contraindication to Long-Term OAC or DOAC**
Gastrointestinal	• History of gastric antral venous ectasia • History of arteriovenous malformations • Gastrointestinal bleeding requiring transfusion (major when >4 U PRBC required) • Ulcerative disease, ulcerative colitis, Crohn disease • Diverticular disease causing recurrent lower gastrointestinal bleeding
Hepatic	• Cirrhosis • Labile INR due to liver dysfunction in patient on warfarin • Thrombocytopenia related to cirrhosis • Persistent atrial fibrillation in cirrhosis
Chronic renal disease	• CKD III-V due to unfavorable metabolism of novel oral anticoagulants • ESRD on hemodialysis • Patients following renal transplant (drug interactions and frequent renal biopsies)
Hematologic	• Treatment with ibrutinib • Von Willebrand's disorder with frequent bleeding events • Hemorrhagic hereditary telangiectasias (Osler Weber Rendu) • Immune thrombocytopenic purpura • Chronic anemias with transfusion requirements
Neurologic	• History of Parkinson disease • Previous stroke with significant disability, related fall risks • Frequent falls (related to tremor, previous stroke, peripheral neuropathy, autonomic neuropathy) • Seizure disorders
Frailty	• Frequent falls • Unstable gait • Drug metabolism issues (age related) • Unable to maintain reliable NOAC adherence
Lifestyle considerations	• High-risk occupations (law enforcement, paratrooper, roofing, high-voltage electrical line workers, firefighters)

Abbreviations: CKD III–V, chronic kidney disease III–V; DOAC, direct oral anticoagulation; ESRD, end-stage renal disease; INR, international normalized ratio; OAC, oral anticoagulation; NOAC, new oral anticoagulant; PRBC, packed red blood cells.

Table 2
Left atrial appendage closure device options and patient selection considerations

LAAC Device	Implant Success	Device Leak Rate (Incomplete LAAC)	Embolization Risk (%)	Device-Related Thrombus (%)	Post-Implant Drug Regimen
Watchman 2.5 (Boston Scientific) FDA approved	>98%	0.3% (>5 mm) 7.9% (1–5 mm)	0.3–0.6	3.7	• Warfarin 45 d plus ASA, then DAPT until 6 mo, then ASA alone
Watchman FLX (Boston Scientific) NCT02702271	>98%	N/A	N/A	N/A	• DOAC 45d with ASA, DAPT 6 mo, then ASA alone long term
Amulet (Abbott Medical) NCT02879448	>96%	7.1% (1–5 mm)	0.2–0.7	1.7–3.1	• Antiplatelet therapy (DAPT) 6 mo, then ASA alone
LARIAT (SentreHEART) NCT02513797	High (no RCT)	10%–21% (1–5 mm)	None	<1 (rare)	• Antiplatelet therapy (off-label use) • 1 y DOAC or OAC (Amaze Trial)
Atriclip (Atricure)	High (no RCT)	1%–4% (malposition, large stump)	None	<1% (rare)	• Antiplatelet therapy (off-label use)

Abbreviations: DOAC, direct oral anticoagulation; OAC, oral anticoagulation; N/A, not applicable; RCT, randomized clinical trial.
Data from Refs.[28–30]

Patients with known resistance to clopidogrel or a true aspirin allergy should be counseled on the potential for higher risk for adverse events, and potentially not undergo an endocardial device-based approach. Allergy testing and aspirin desensitization has been used to overcome this barrier, although it will often delay LAAC implantation for many months. Also, it is notable that an allergy to nickel is a contraindication to LAAC with an endocardial nitinol-based occluder (Watchman, Watchman FLX, Amulet). In select cases we have sent patients for formal nickel allergy testing to clarify their risk, although the results of this strategy in improving patient outcome have not been demonstrated.

Absolute Contraindications to Anticoagulation

When intolerance to anticoagulation is considered "absolute" (ie, active subdural hematoma, subarachnoid hemorrhage, intraparenchymal bleed, cerebral amyloid angiopathy, or active critical bleeding into an organ or critical space), then the above regimen needs to be altered. The ASAP-TOO clinical trial is ongoing and can help provide formal data, the ASAP registry and recent EWOLUTION registry data support that, for most cases, an antiplatelet regimen alone can suffice for post-implant drug regimen with a minor uptick in DRT rate.[20,21] Inherent to the population being implanted with Watchman, many patients may be deemed suitable for short-term anticoagulation, yet major adverse bleeding recurs during the 6 to 12 weeks post-implant. In most instances, DOAC or warfarin is stopped, and the underlying bleed is addressed before attempting any continued blood thinner. This may potentially increase the risk of DRT formation although it has not been scientifically studied.

In 2013, the ASAP registry was performed with the intent to determine the safety of LAAC in patients who are ineligible for warfarin therapy. One hundred and fifty patients with NVAF and an average CHADS2 and CHA2DS2VASc score of 2.8 and 4.4, respectively, were included in the study. Mean follow-up was approximately 14 months, and the ischemic stroke rate determined at the end of the study was 7.3%. This was lower than the expected stroke rate according to the stroke risk stratification scores (CHADS2 and CHADS2Vasc) mentioned above.[20] Similarly the EWOLUTION trial enrolled 1025 patients, 83% of whom were treated with antiplatelet therapy alone, whereas only 8% were treated with warfarin. The overall ischemic stroke rate was 1.1% annually.[21]

Ongoing studies including, PINNACLE-FLX, ASAP-TOO, and the Amulet versus Watchman IDE trial (see **Table 2**) all will give more information if DOAC short term, or simply DAPT, will be safe after Watchman, Watchman FLX, or Amulet. In addition, in patients who cannot tolerate OAC, DOAC, or antiplatelet therapy, the subxiphoid LARIAT (SentreHEART, Redwood City, CA), or a stand-alone Atriclip (Atricure, West Chester, OH), could prove to be most reasonable option (**Table 3**), as neither OAC nor antiplatelet therapies are required. Although we say this often, we should remember that, in the initial LARIAT trial, the fine print documents that at 1 year, we believe that most patients had been treated at some time with an anticoagulant. Despite biological plausibility and good registry data, there are no prospective clinical trials to date supporting these epicardial approaches as an AF stroke prevention strategy.

One consideration in LAAC is DRT, which occurs not infrequently and requires anticoagulation treatment if diagnosed on follow-up TEEs. In the EWOLUTION trial, DRT was observed in 28 patients (3.7%) but was not correlated with antiplatelet versus warfarin therapy.[22] Similarly, in both the PROTECT AF and ASAP studies there was approximately a 4% DRT risk, which resulted in 1.5% stroke rate.[9] It should be noted that DAPT will not effectively treat DRT, and that OAC or DOAC would need to be resumed in these patients for adequate therapy at least for a short time, thus placing those patients at increased risk of complications intended to be avoided by performing LAAC and discontinuing OAC in the first place.

In summary, consideration for patient selection for LAAC should be based on both a balance of the current attributed NVAF-related stroke risk for the patient, the acute procedure risk, and the post-implant drug regimen selection. Consultation with neurology or neurosurgery can be helpful when considering LAAC shortly after an intracranial bleed. These are patients in whom a 30-day or inpatient mortality risk can approach greater than 35%, and early resumption of DOAC/OAC is associated with improved outcomes.[23,24]

Table 3
Clinical trials ongoing for left atrial appendage closure devices expanding indications

Device Trial	AF Population	Subjects (n)	Primary Endpoint	Enrolment Status (Sept 2019)
PINNACLE-FLX (Watchman FLX) NCT02702271	CHADS 2 Vasc 3 or higher and Watchman 2.5 candidate	458	Seal of LAA by TEE at 45 d and 1 y, device leak <5 mm	Closed (October 2018)
Amulet vs Watchman (Amulet IDE) NCT02879448	CHADS 2 Vasc 3 or higher Watchman 2.5 candidate	1878	Stroke or systemic embolism at 18 mo, device leak <5 mm	Closed (March 8, 2019)
OPTION trial (Watchman FLX) NCT03795298	Patient undergoing paroxysmal or persistent AF ablation	1600	Stroke, all-cause death, and embolism at 36 mo	Ongoing Opened in 2019
AMAZE trial (LARIAT) NCT02513797	Persistent or longstanding symptomatic AF	600	Recurrence of AF/ AT >30 s on 12 mo Holter	Ongoing (535 subjects to date)
Wavecrest vs Watchman (Wavecrest) NCT03302494	CHADS 2 Vasc 3 or higher Watchman 2.5 candidate	1250	Death, major bleeding, or ischemic stroke at 24 mo	Ongoing Opened in 2019

Abbreviations: AF, atrial fibrillation; AT, atrial tachyarrhythmia; LAA, left atrial appendage; TEE, transesophageal echocardiography.

Treatment Failure of Anticoagulation or Lifelong Anticoagulation Indicated for Alternate Diagnosis

An additional group that could qualify for LAAC are those who have been adequately treated with OAC or DOAC, but in whom LAA thrombus develops, or an ischemic stroke occurs in the setting of AF with a PFO while on anticoagulation. These patients may be optimally suited to undergo LAAC as they could tolerate peri-procedure anticoagulation (no previous major bleeding). In fact, there could be consideration for some patients at high risk to remain on anticoagulation long term after LAAC. A potential unproven "double coverage" against embolic stroke risk.

Clearly excluded from consideration for LAAC referral to replace anticoagulation would be patients with thrombus on a mechanical heart valve, left ventricular assist device recipients, or a patient with a left ventricular thrombus in the setting of severe LV failure who has suffered an embolic stroke. However, patients with AF and a hypercoagulable state (Factor V Leiden, Prothrombin 20210 gene mutation, Protein C or S deficiency, or antiphospholipid antibodies), history of heparin-induced thrombocytopenia, deep venous thrombosis, or pulmonary emboli, may identify additional double coverage patients, knowing that the post-implant drug regimen would still include lifelong ongoing anticoagulation. The inevitability of temporary cessation of anticoagulation for these patients, particularly if stuck in persistent AF, places them at high stroke risk. This is a cohort of patients warranting future study, and a hypercoagulable work-up before LAAC could provide insight into patients at increased risk for DRT.[25]

Role for Patient Preference

As described above, the initial studies for LAAC were compared head to head with warfarin, which proved noninferiority. Front-line therapy randomized trials with LAAC head to head versus DOAC or OAC in all comers with NVAF are needed (CHADS2Vasc score 2 or higher in men, 3 or higher in women). This could move LAAC to a direct-to-patient therapy where patients would be able to make an informed choice to undergo LAAC closure for NVAF, rather than indefinitely be on oral anticoagulation up front. Many patients will factor in convenience, long-term drug cost, their own ability to comply with international normalized ratio testing, diet restrictions, or drug dosing and reduced risk of drug-drug interactions into their decisions. This is an important one and will become even more so as we develop more data.

Patients Who May Not Be Candidates for Left Atrial Appendage Closure

In addition to the patients with low stroke risk (CHAD2DS2VASc <2), there are a variety of patients who may not be appropriate for referral for LAAC. Firstly, patients with specific cardiac anatomy may not qualify for LAAC. As described above, those with advanced valvular AF would not qualify for LAAC (or NOACs) and should be managed with warfarin. Surgical LAA ligation, clipping, or excision should be performed if a patient with severe valve disease undergoes open chest valve repair. Minimally invasive LAA clipping during nonsternotomy approach to aortic or mitral valve replacement is effective, but epicardial LAA suture ligation through a thoracoscopic approach can be challenging. In a large registry analysis of the Society of Thoracic Surgeons data, patients who underwent LAA occlusion had a significant reduction in mortality and embolic events.[26] Referral for LAA closure at the time of valve surgery or AF surgery (concomitant Cox-Maze procedure) is recommended in guidelines (IIa recommendation).[27]

Patients with challenging LAA anatomy (broad cauliflower shape), large ostia greater than 31 mm, difficult LAA dimensions restricted by limited depth, or persistent clot in LAA may prohibit use of currently available LAAC devices. Severely reduced LVEF may also disqualify a patient from LAAC with Watchman. Patients with limited life expectancy (typically <1 year) should not be referred for LAAC and rather should be managed medically. At present, patients who cannot tolerate any form of anticoagulation/antiplatelet therapy do not qualify for Watchman device due to the need for short-term anticoagulation both before and after device placement although, as described above, this indication may change soon with the data taken from ASAP-TOO and the Amulet IDE trials.

CURRENT INVESTIGATIONS

Patients, particularly those with absolute contraindications to OAC or NOAC, may wish to consider enrolment in IDE clinical trials, or trials for LAA closure in the setting of larger considerations in treating their AF. Amulet, Lariat, and Atriclip devices all available, but typically require the institution be involved in the clinical studies. As described above, the LARIAT may be particularly attractive in patients who cannot receive any anticoagulation; however, the AMAZE clinical trial is looking at AF recurrence postablation, and not embolic stroke risk, as the primary endpoint.

SUMMARY

Left atrial appendage closure as an alternative to long-term anticoagulation in patients with NVAF and a suitable rationale to consider Watchman LAAC casts a fairly broad net. We review the specifics for the indications, FDA labeling, and CMS coverage, as well as patients who clearly should be excluded from consideration of LAAC. Patients with unique scenarios in which LAAC could provide benefit over no therapy, or in addition to lifelong anticoagulation, are an intriguing population that warrants further ongoing study. LAAC remains a class IIb recommendation in the setting of relative intolerance to anticoagulation, and several large randomized trials nearing completion could support moving LAAC up in the guidelines.

DISCLOSURE

Consulting and Advisory Board; (All <$10,000 per annum); Boston Scientific Inc, Abbott Medical Inc, Medtronic Inc Research funding; Investigator Initiated studies (funding paid to Vanderbilt University Medical Center); Boston Scientific Inc, Medtronic Inc, Atricure Inc, Boehringer-Ingelheim Pharmaceuticals Inc (C.R. Ellis). No disclosures (G.G. Jackson).

REFERENCES

1. Gage BF, Waterman AD, Shannon W, et al. Validation of clinical classification schemes for predicting stroke: results from the National Registry of Atrial Fibrillation. JAMA 2001;285(22):2864–70.
2. Olesen JB, Torp-Pedersen C, Hansen ML, et al. The value of the CHA2DS2-VASc score for refining stroke risk stratification in patients with atrial fibrillation with a CHADS2 score 0–1: a nationwide cohort study. Thromb Haemost 2012;107(6):1172–9.
3. Connolly SJ, Ezekowitz MD, Yusuf S, et al. Dabigatran versus warfarin in patients with atrial fibrillation. N Engl J Med 2009;361(12):1139–51.
4. Patel MR, Mahaffey KW, Garg J, et al. Rivaroxaban versus warfarin in nonvalvular atrial fibrillation. N Engl J Med 2011;365(10):883–91.
5. Giugliano RP, Ruff CT, Baunwald E, et al. Edoxaban versus warfarin in patients with atrial fibrillation. N Engl J Med 2013;369(22):2093–104.
6. Granger CB, Alexander JH, McMurray JJ, et al. Apixaban versus warfarin in patients with atrial fibrillation. N Engl J Med 2011;365(11):981–2.
7. Hsu JC, Maddox TM, Kennedy KF, et al. Oral anticoagulant therapy prescription in patients with atrial fibrillation across the spectrum of stroke risk: insights from the NCDR PINNACLE registry. JAMA Cardiol 2016;1(1):55–62.
8. Yaghi S, Song C, Gray WA, et al. Left atrial appendage function and stroke risk. Stroke 2015; 46(12):3554–9.
9. Holmes DR Jr, Kar S, Price MJ, et al. Prospective randomized evaluation of the Watchman left atrial appendage closure device in patients with atrial fibrillation versus long-term warfarin therapy: the PREVAIL trial. J Am Coll Cardiol 2014;64(1):1–12.
10. Holmes DR, Reddy VY, Turi ZG, et al. Percutaneous closure of the left atrial appendage versus warfarin therapy for prevention of stroke in patients with atrial fibrillation: a randomised non-inferiority trial. Lancet 2009;374(9689):534–42.
11. Centers for Medicare & Medicaid Services. Decision memo for percutaneous left atrial appendage (LAA) closure therapy (CAG-00445N). 2016. Available at: https://www.cms.gov/medicare-coverage-database/details/nca-decision-memo.aspx?NCAId=281&ExpandComments=n&DocID=CAG-00445N&bc=gAAAAAgAAgAAAA%3d%3d&.
12. U.S. Food and Drug Administration. Watchman LAA closure technology—P130013 [Internet] Silver Spring (MD): U.S. Food and Drug Administration. 2015. Available at: https://www.accessdata.fda.gov/cdrh_docs/pdf13/p130013a.pdf. Accessed August 21, 2019.
13. January CT, Wann LS, Calkins H, et al. 2019 AHA/ACC/HRS focused update of the 2014 AHA/ACC/HRS guideline for the management of patients with atrial fibrillation. Heart Rhythm 2019;16(8):e66–93.
14. Dukkipati SR, Kar S, Holmes DR Jr, et al. Device-related thrombus after left atrial appendage closure: incidence, predictors, and outcomes. Circulation 2018;138(9):874–85.
15. Alkhouli M, Busu T, Shah K, et al. Incidence and clinical impact of device-related thrombus following percutaneous left atrial appendage occlusion: a meta-analysis. JACC Clin Electrophysiol 2018;4: 1629–37.
16. Hutt E, Wazni OM, Kaur S, et al. Left atrial appendage closure device implantation in patients at very high risk for stroke. Heart Rhythm 2019. https://doi.org/10.1016/j.hrthm.2019.07.011.
17. Eikelboom JW, Connolly SJ, Brueckmann M, et al. Dabigatran versus warfarin in patients with mechanical heart valves. N Engl J Med 2013;369(13): 1206–14.
18. Bergmann MW, Betts TR, Sievert H, et al. Safety and efficacy of early anticoagulation drug regimens after WATCHMAN left atrial appendage closure: three-month data from the EWOLUTION prospective, multicentre, monitored international WATCHMAN LAA closure registry. EuroIntervention 2017;13(7):877–84.
19. Enomoto Y, Gadiyaram VK, Gianni C, et al. Use of non-warfarin oral anticoagulants instead of warfarin during left atrial appendage closure with the Watchman device. Heart Rhythm 2017;14(1):19–24.

20. Reddy VY, Möbius-Winkler S, Miller MA, et al. Left atrial appendage closure with the Watchman device in patients with a contraindication for oral anticoagulation: the ASAP study (ASA Plavix Feasibility study with Watchman left atrial appendage closure technology). J Am Coll Cardiol 2013;61:2551–6.

21. Bergmann MW, Ince H, Kische S, et al. Real-world safety and efficacy of WATCHMAN LAA closure at one year in patients on dual antiplatelet therapy: results of the DAPT subgroup from the EWOLUTION all-comers study. EuroIntervention 2018;(13): 2003–11.

22. Boersma LV, Ince H, Kische S, et al. Efficacy and safety of left atrial appendage closure with WATCHMAN in patients with or without contraindication to oral anticoagulation: 1-year follow-up outcome data of the EWOLUTION trial. Heart Rhythm 2017;14:1302–8.

23. Perreault S, Côté R, White-Guay B, et al. Anticoagulants in older patients with nonvalvular atrial fibrillation after intracranial hemorrhage. J Stroke 2019; 21(2):195–206.

24. Inohara T, Xian Y, Liang L, et al. Association of intracerebral hemorrhage among patients taking non-vitamin K antagonist vs vitamin K antagonist oral anticoagulants with in-hospital mortality. JAMA 2018; 319(5):463–73.

25. Berge E, Haug KB, Sandset EC, et al. The factor V Leiden, prothrombin gene 20210GA, methylenetetrahydrofolate reductase 677CT and platelet glycoprotein IIIa 1565TC mutations in patients with acute ischemic stroke and atrial fibrillation. Stroke 2007;38(3):1069–71.

26. Friedman DJ, Piccini JP, Wang T, et al. Association between left atrial appendage occlusion and readmission for thromboembolism among patients with atrial fibrillation undergoing concomitant cardiac surgery. JAMA 2018;319:365–74.

27. Badhwar V, Rankin JS, Damino RJ, et al. The Society of Thoracic Surgeons 2016 clinical practice guidelines for the surgical treatment of atrial fibrillation. Ann Thorac Surg 2017;103:329–41.

28. Landmesser U, Tondo C, Camm J, et al. Left atrial appendage occlusion with the AMPLATZER Amulet device: one-year follow-up from the prospective global Amulet observational registry. EuroIntervention 2018;14(5):e590–7.

29. Alkhouli M, Busu T, Shah K, et al. Incidence and impact of DRT following percutaneous LAAO. JACC Clin EP 2018;4(12):1629–37.

30. Boersma LV, Ince H, Kische S, et al. Evaluating real-world clinical outcomes in atrial fibrillation patients receiving the WATCHMAN left atrial appendage closure technology. Circ Arrhythm Electrophysiol 2019;12(4):e006841.

Anatomic Considerations for Epicardial and Endocardial Left Atrial Appendage Closure

Aleksandr Voskoboinik, MBBS, PhD, Randall J. Lee, MD, PhD*

KEYWORDS

• Left atrial appendage • Isolation • Ligation • Amplatzer amulet occluder • Watchman • LARIAT
• AtriClip

KEY POINTS

• Preprocedural imaging, including transesophageal echocardiography and computed tomography, is critical to planning the most appropriate means of achieving left atrial appendage closure.
• It is vital to accurately assess left atrial appendage morphology, including ostial width, landing zone, and depth, to plan the most appropriate approach and device size.

INTRODUCTION

As the primary source of emboli in approximately 90% of patients with nonvalvular atrial fibrillation (AF), closure of the left atrial appendage (LAA) is a widely accepted treatment strategy for patients with contraindications to anticoagulation. The LAA may also be the source of focal tachycardias and is potentially important in the maintenance of persistent AF, with electrical isolation an increasingly adopted antiarrhythmic strategy. Once a decision has been made to close the LAA, preprocedural planning is critical to ensure appropriate device selection based on patient and anatomic factors. Important considerations include LAA size, morphology, and orientation for planning of transseptal puncture if an endocardial approach is to be undertaken. Current commercially available endocardial closure devices are the Watchman (Boston Scientific) and Amplatzer Amulet (Abbott), whereas epicardial systems include the LARIAT (SentreHEART) and AtriClip (AtriCure) systems.

Anatomically, the LAA is usually directed anterosuperiorly, and arises from the lateral and anterior left atrial wall. It overlaps the pulmonary trunk or right ventricular outflow tract (left border) as well as the left main or circumflex coronary artery with its lower surface overlying the left ventricle[1] (**Fig. 1**). However, it is important to be aware of anatomic variants that may pose challenges for closure, including an LAA tip that is directed backward and laterally or passes behind the aorta and pulmonary trunk to reside in the transverse pericardial sinus. The Coumadin ridge separates the LAA orifice from the orifices of the left pulmonary veins; however, the level and distance between the LAA and pulmonary vein is variable. The LAA orifice is separated from the mitral annulus by the smooth muscular wall of the left atrial vestibule. Patients may have between 1 and 4 LAA lobes, and morphologies include the so-called chicken wing (48%), windsock (19%), cactus (30%), and cauliflower (3%),[2] as shown in **Fig. 2**.

PREPROCEDURAL PLANNING

Several factors influence whether an endocardial or epicardial approach is taken. Endocardial occlusion devices require the ability to safely achieve

Department of Electrophysiology, University of California San Francisco, 500 Parnassus Ave., MU-East Fourth Floor, San Francisco, CA 94143, USA
* Corresponding author.
E-mail address: Randall.Lee@ucsf.edu

Card Electrophysiol Clin 12 (2020) 39–45
https://doi.org/10.1016/j.ccep.2019.11.001
1877-9182/20/© 2019 Elsevier Inc. All rights reserved.

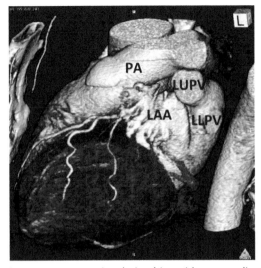

Fig. 1. LAA: anatomic relationships with surrounding structures. LLPV, left lower pulmonary vein; LUPV, left upper pulmonary vein; PA, pulmonary artery.

transseptal access (may be contraindicated with prior septal occlusion devices), suitable LAA anatomy (to ensure a proper seal), and a period of antithrombotic therapy (until complete endothelialization of the occluder occurs). This period of antithrombotic therapy is variable. In European and Asian countries, LAA occlusion with an endocardial device is most commonly performed in patients in whom there is either a relative or absolute contraindication to anticoagulation. In these patients, more typically only antiplatelet therapy is given.[3]

Epicardial systems do not require a period of postprocedure anticoagulation however, pericardial adhesions impede mobility within the pericardial space and hence the LARIAT device is contraindicated in patients with prior cardiac surgery or severe pericarditis. Severe obesity,

epicardial ablation, uremia, and pectus excavatum are also relative contraindications because of challenges with pericardial access and/or pericardial adhesions.[4]

The following features make deployment of endocardial closure devices particularly challenging[5]:

1. Retroflex chicken-wing bends characterized by a short LAA ostium followed by a 180° turn with the ongoing lobe traversing behind the pulmonary artery. Surgical clipping may be the only option for this particular anatomy.
2. Short LAA depth with early bifurcations.
3. Unusual protruding pectinate muscles and/or ridge.
4. Very close proximity to surrounding structures such as left upper pulmonary vein and mitral annulus, particularly with lobe and disc designs that may cause partial obstruction.

A preprocedural computed tomography (CT) scan and/or transesophageal echocardiography (TEE) are critical for assessment of LAA size, morphology, and orientation because of the significant variability in anatomy. Important measurements include LAA ostium size (width), width of landing zone (neck), and LAA depth, and it is also important to assess for LAA thrombus (**Fig. 3**). CT images with three-dimensional (3D) reconstruction provide a particularly useful representation of LAA morphology and enable visualization of proximity to surrounding structures. LAA measurements should be performed when the appendage is at its largest at the conclusion of ventricular systole to avoid device undersizing. In addition, hypovolemia is important to avoid because the dimensions of the LAA may vary. To optimize placement, a left atrial pressure of greater than 12 mmHg should be obtained. Eccentric LAA ostia or lobes originating close to the ostium may

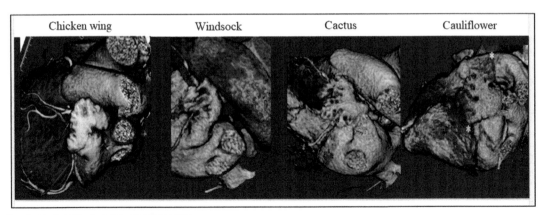

Fig. 2. Variability in LAA morphologies.

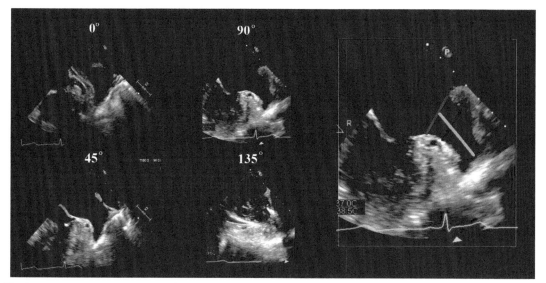

Fig. 3. LAA assessment using 4 angles, and measurement of LAA ostium width (*red*), LAA landing zone (*blue*), and LAA depth (*green*).

increase the risk of incomplete seal and peridevice leak. A thin-walled ostium, neck, and/or lobe increase perforation risk. A cone-shaped appendage with a progressive increase in dimensions from tip to orifice may transmit compressive forces, pushing the device out of the LAA and resulting in migration or embolization. Severe angulation between the neck and ostium may also present technical challenges.[6]

Awareness of surrounding structures is important, because the device may impinge on the left upper pulmonary vein or mitral annulus and there have also been rare case reports of device erosion into the left circumflex artery and pulmonary artery. The left phrenic nerve also overlays the LAA as it runs along the pericardial surface. CT scans may provide estimates of dimensions that are 2 to 3 mm larger than on two-dimensional TEE and 2 mm larger than 3D TEE.[1,7]

The gold standard for periprocedural imaging of the LAA is TEE, which may be contraindicated in the setting of esophageal disease (eg, esophagectomy, varices). TEE enables multiplanar views at various angles to scan through the appendage and is able to guide positioning of endocardial devices and assess for leaks around the device using color Doppler. Intracardiac echocardiography (ICE) avoids esophageal intubation and does not require general anesthesia, but provides only limited 45° LAA views, which may be overcome by either advancing the ICE probe into the left atrium via the transseptal puncture or imaging the LAA from the right ventricular outflow tract.[7] Angiography also provides adjunctive information. The LAA ostium is best visible on right anterior oblique (RAO) cranial views (RAO 30°, cranial 20°) and RAO caudal views (RAO 30°, caudal 20°).[8]

Watchman

Endocardial occlusion can be achieved using the Watchman closure device, which contains a self-expanding nitinol frame with fixation barbs and a 160-μm polyethylene membrane covering the left atrial device surface. There are 5 available sizes (**Table 1**) and, to ensure stable positioning, a size greater than 10% to 20% of the LAA diameter (width) is preferred. The largest LAA ostial measurement is used to select the size of the Watchman device.[9]

It is important to characterize LAA morphology because this may affect ease of implant, because it is critical to ensure there is adequate depth to deploy the device. A windsock morphology with 1 dominant lobe and adequate depth represents the most straightforward anatomy. Challenges may be encountered with a chicken-wing LAA if the proximal portion (before the sharp bend) is shorter than the maximum LAA ostium width and a cauliflower LAA with several lobes to cover and limited depth at the bifurcation of the lobes.[10,11]

It is critical to assess LAA morphology and measure LAA ostium width and depth in 4 views on TEE (0°, 45°, 90°, 135°) with the device chosen based on maximum LAA ostium width. Because of the oval shape of the ostium, larger LAA ostial diameters are often obtained in the 120° to 135° planes. The LAA depth must be as long as the LAA ostium

Table 1
Sizing of watchman device based on left atrial appendage ostium width

Maximum LAA Ostium Width (mm)	Device Size (mm)	Deployed Diameter, 80%–92% of Original (mm)
17–19	21	16.8–19.3
20–22	24	19.2–22.1
23–25	27	21.6–24.8
26–28	30	24.0–27.6
29–31	33	26.4–30.4

width. The ideal location for transseptal puncture is the midinferior aspect of the posterior septum, which directs the sheath toward the LAA, which is located superiorly and anteriorly, thereby enabling coaxial deployment of the device. An exception to this general transseptal puncture position is when the LAA orifice is oriented superiorly as in a reverse chicken wing.[11,12] A transseptal puncture in the most anterior aspect of the foramen in this setting is most advantageous to orient an anterior shaped sheath to deliver the Watchman device coaxial into the LAA.

Criteria for deployment include:

1. Positioning at or slightly distal to the LAA ostium
2. Device spans the entire LAA ostium and seals the LAA from the left atrium, with all lobes distal to the device (jet around the device, <5 mm)
3. Implant stability (tug test to ensure the LAA and Watchman move in unison)

Fig. 4 shows a successfully deployed Watchman device with minimal jet around the device.

Amplatzer Amulet

The Amplatzer Amulet is a self-expanding endocardial LAA occlusion device made of nitinol mesh with a disc-and-lobe configuration. The proximal disc is 6 to 7 mm wider than the distal lobe and seals the LAA ostium, whereas the distal

lobe anchors the device to the LAA landing zone (body or neck) using stabilizing wires. A waist connects the lobe and disc.[13]

Sizes range from 16 to 34 mm, and are appropriate for landing-zone diameters from 11 to 31 mm. Sizing depends on the widest landing zone as assessed by CT, TEE, or angiography. The device size should be greater than or equal to 2 mm wider than the (widest) LAA landing zone diameter and is usually implanted ~12 mm inside the LAA cavity.[14] As such, the Amulet can accommodate shallow LAA placement, because only 10 mm in depth is required for deployment. It is also well suited for larger LAAs, with 31-mm and 34-mm sizes available. The posteroinferior septum is also the ideal location for transseptal puncture; however a more anterior puncture may be preferred for reverse-chicken-wing anatomy with a more anterior ostium.[15,16]

Criteria for successful deployment include:

1. Adequate apposition of the distal lobe to the LAA wall
2. Good seal as shown by a concave shape of the proximal disc
3. Separation between the proximal disc and distal lobe
4. Distal lobe in the axis of the LAA landing zone
5. Lobe positioned distal to the left circumflex on TEE (at least two-thirds)
6. Implant stability (tug test)

A sandwich technique may be used in patients with a chicken-wing appendage characterized by a bend in the proximal or middle aspect of the dominant LAA lobe with a short neck. In this situation, a larger device is often required and its lobe is implanted parallel to the length of the LAA wing (body), thereby sandwiching the LAA ostium between the device's disc and lobe. Disc-and-lobe devices that are oversized may impinge on surrounding structures, such as the left upper pulmonary vein and mitral annulus.[16]

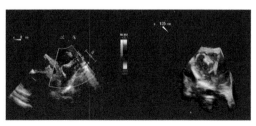

Fig. 4. Successfully deployed device (two-dimensional view with color Doppler and 3D).

LARIAT

The LARIAT suture delivery device requires a combined endocardial and epicardial approach for LAA ligation. It involves advancing a magnetic tip wire endocardially after transept catheterization into the most anterior lobe of the LAA, which meets a second magnetic tip wire coaxially in the pericardial space, which must be accessed via an anterior pericardial approach.[17] The ideal transseptal position to allow the wires to meet coaxially is the mid to lower height, aiming for a mid to posterior puncture (a higher puncture or puncture via a patent foramen ovale directs the sheath toward the left pulmonary veins, rather than the anterior aspect of the LAA as desired). The LARIAT snare is then advanced over the wires via the epicardial sheath and tightened.[18]

It is important to assess the maximum LAA width with CT angiography and TEE (best in 135° view). The first-generation LARIAT was restricted to an LAA width of 40 mm (the device's loop must negotiate a fixed diameter when snaring the LAA); however, the snare width was increased to 50 mm with the newest-generation LARIAT.[19] Other anatomic contraindications include any LAA morphology that travels behind the pulmonary artery. A bilobed (or multilobed) LAA with lobes oriented in different angles and a posteriorly rotated heart can be more difficult to close with the LARIAT, but this can be achieved with careful manipulation of the LARIAT.[20]

CT angiography also facilitates planning of pericardial access, with the anteroposterior (AP) view of the CT guiding the direction of the needle toward the LAA and the lateral view providing information about the most inferior aspect of the sternum and the space between the sternum and anterior surface of the heart, and directing the steepness of the needle.

An anterior pericardial approach (**Fig. 5**) is undertaken using a telescopic approach with a micropuncture needle (needle-in-needle approach). In an AP projection, the needle should be directed lateral to the LAA (which is lateral to the pulmonary artery), thus the pulmonary artery silhouette and pulmonary vasculature hilum may be used as landmarks and the needle directed toward the left shoulder just lateral to these landmarks, entering the pericardial space 1 to 2 cm above the apex. Pericardial access that is directed medially does not allow the LARIAT to be directed posteriorly toward the LAA. The proper orientation of pericardial access is toward the lateral aspect of the pulmonary hilum, which is directed toward the LAA and allows the LARIAT to be directed posteriorly to capture the LAA.[18]

The 90° left lateral view confirms that the pericardial space is entered anteriorly (as shown by the direction of the wire in **Fig. 5**B). As the guidewire is advanced out of the needle, it is important to check in the left anterior oblique (LAO) fluoroscopic view that the guidewire outlines the left heart border and loops around the pericardial space crossing the midline (to confirm that the wire is not in the right ventricle and pulmonary artery). Once it is confirmed that the wire is in the pericardial space, a sheath can be inserted.

The endocardial magnet-tipped guidewire is inserted into the anterior and superior aspect of the LAA, and this is confirmed by either 30° RAO or 20° caudal fluoroscopic orientations as well as TEE. The epicardial magnet-tipped wire is then passed through the epicardial sheath using the 30° LAO and RAO caudal fluoroscopic views to ensure the magnets connect and symmetrically align (**Fig. 6**) to provide a monorail for the LARIAT device directing the snare from the anterior cardiac surface posteriorly toward the LAA.[19]

Correct snare orientation is confirmed in 30° LAO projection when the radio-opaque marker on the distal end of the LARIAT is on the left side and the snare legs are parallel, with the snare able to move freely over the posterior aspect of the LAA. Under TEE guidance, a balloon catheter is then inflated at the mouth of the LAA and the snare is closed over a balloon (**Fig. 7**). The suture

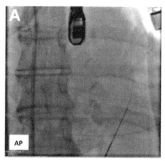
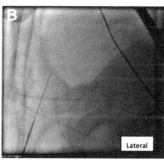

Fig. 5. An anterior pericardial approach in AP (*A*) and 90° left lateral (*B*) views. The wire enters the pericardial space anteriorly, which is critical to maneuvering the suture delivery device over the anterior surface of the right ventricle toward the tip of the LAA in its most anterior aspect.

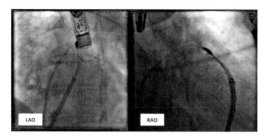

Fig. 6. Correct alignment of the snare over the LAA.

is only released when contrast left atrial angiography and TEE (lack of color flow on Doppler) confirm complete LAA closure. Potential advantages of the LARIAT compared with endocardial devices include negligible risk of embolization or device erosion, antiarrhythmic effects of electrical isolation of the LAA, and lower risk of residual leak. However, risks associated with pericardial access (eg, right ventricular laceration/perforation) exist, whereas risk of LAA perforation exists for all approaches.[20]

AtriClip

The AtriClip is a purely epicardial LAA occlusion device composed of 2 parallel titanium tubes with nitinol springs acting as a self-closing clamp. It can be applied during cardiac surgery or thoracoscopically via the left chest.[21] It requires the ability to perform single-lung ventilation. Significant pericardial adhesions may also pose challenges. However, it may be the only option in patients with a retropulmonic LAA or patients unable to undergo transseptal

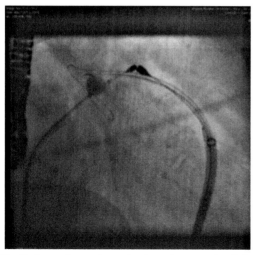

Fig. 7. Snare located proximal to the mouth of the LAA (marked by a balloon catheter) to confirm complete LAA closure.

puncture and/or an endocardial approach.[22] The AtriClip is not restricted by LAA ostial size or LAA anatomy/morphology. During a thoracoscopic approach, the phrenic nerve is identified and an incision is made 1 cm below to identify 2the LAA. The base of the LAA is then assessed for size (range, 35–50 mm) and an AtriClip then applied. The procedure can only be performed by cardiac surgeons and long-term follow-up data are lacking. However, rates of incomplete ligation with remnant stumps (posing a risk of thrombus formation) are lower than for stapling or suture ligation (endocardial or epicardial).[23]

SUMMARY

An in-depth understanding of each patients' LAA anatomy is critical before proceeding with occlusion. Preprocedural TEE and CT angiography provide complimentary information to guide decision making. Once LAA morphology, width, and depth are assessed in conjunction with other patient factors, a decision can be made regarding suitability for endocardial or epicardial closure. With each approach, periprocedural imaging with TEE, fluoroscopy, and angiography facilitate safe and effective transseptal puncture and/or pericardial access, as well as deployment of devices to ensure complete occlusion without residual leak.

DISCLOSURE

Dr A. Voskoboinik has received fellowship support from Boston Scientific and Abbott Medical. Dr R.J. Lee is a consultant and equity holder in Sentre-HEART/AtriCure.

REFERENCES

1. Beigel R, Wunderlich NC, Ho SY, et al. The left atrial appendage: anatomy, function, and noninvasive evaluation. JACC Cardiovasc Imaging 2014;7(12): 1251–65.
2. Freixa X, Tzikas A, Basmadjian A, et al. The chicken-enwing morphology: an anatomical challenge for left atrial appendage occlusion. J Interv Cardiol 2013;26:509–14.
3. Blackshear JL, Odell JA. Appendage obliteration to reduce stroke in cardiac surgical patients with atrial fibrillation. Ann Thorac Surg 1996;61(2):755–9.
4. Aryana A, Singh SM, Doshi SK, et al. Advances in left atrial appendage occlusion strategies. J Atr Fibrillation 2013;6(4):929.
5. Di Biase L, Santangeli P, Anselmino M, et al. Does the left atrial appendage morphology correlate with the risk of stroke in patients with atrial fibrillation?

Results from a multicenter study. J Am Coll Cardiol 2012;60:531–8.

6. Patti G, Pengo V, Marcucci R, et al. The left atrial appendage: from embryology to prevention of thromboembolism. Eur Heart J 2017;38(12):877–87.

7. Wunderlich NC, Beigel R, Swaans MJ, et al. Percutaneous interventions for left atrial appendage exclusion: options, assessment, and imaging using 2D and 3D echocardiography. JACC Cardiovasc Imaging 2015;8(4):472–88.

8. Lin AC, Knight BP. What is the role of left atrial appendage closure in the rhythm control of atrial fibrillation? Curr Treat Options Cardiovasc Med 2018;20(3):24.

9. Möbius-Winkler S, Sandri M, Mangner N, et al. The WATCHMAN left atrial appendage closure device for atrial fibrillation. J Vis Exp 2012;60:3671.

10. Reddy VY, Möbius-Winkler S, Miller MA, et al. Left atrial appendage closure with the Watchman device in patients with a contraindication for oral anticoagulation: the ASAP study (ASA plavix feasibility study with watchman left atrial appendage closure technology). J Am Coll Cardiol 2013;61(25):2551–6.

11. Panaich SS, Munger T, Friedman P, et al. Case-based discussion regarding challenges in patient selection and procedural planning in left atrial appendage occlusion. Mayo Clin Proc 2018;93(5):630–8.

12. Romero J, Natale A, Di Biase LLAA. Morphology and physiology: "the missing piece in the puzzle". J Cardiovasc Electrophysiol 2015;26:928–33.

13. Parashar A, Tuzcu EM, Kapadia SR. Cardiac plug I and amulet devices: left atrial appendage closure for stroke prophylaxis in atrial fibrillation. J Atr Fibrillation 2015;7(6):1236.

14. Tzikas A. Left atrial appendage occlusion with amplatzer cardiac plug and amplatzer amulet: a clinical trials update. J Atr Fibrillation 2017;10(4):1651.

15. Messas N, Ibrahim R. The amplatzer amulet device: technical considerations and procedural approach. Interv Cardiol Clin 2018;7(2):213–8.

16. Tzikas A, Gafoor S, Meerkin D, et al. Left atrial appendage occlusion with the AMPLATZER Amulet device: an expert consensus step-by-step approach. EuroIntervention 2016;11(13):1512–21.

17. Pillarisetti J, Reddy YM, Gunda S, et al. Endocardial (Watchman) vs epicardial (Lariat) left atrial appendage exclusion devices: understanding the differences in the location and type of leaks and their clinical implications. Heart Rhythm 2015;12(7):1501–7.

18. Koneru JN, Badhwar N, Ellenbogen KA, et al. LAA ligation using the LARIAT suture delivery device: tips and tricks for a successful procedure. Heart Rhythm 2014;11(5):911–21.

19. Bartus K, Han FT, Bednarek J, et al. Percutaneous left atrial appendage suture ligation using the LARIAT device in patients with atrial fibrillation: initial clinical experience. J Am Coll Cardiol 2013;62(2):108–18.

20. Srivastava MC, See VY, Dawood MY, et al. A review of the LARIAT device: insights from the cumulative clinical experience. Springerplus 2015;4:522.

21. Bedeir K, Warriner S, Kofsky E, et al. Left atrial appendage epicardial clip (AtriClip): essentials and post-procedure management. J Atr Fibrillation 2019;11(6):2087.

22. Salzberg S, Emmert M. Surgical epicardial left atrial appendage closure: a true alternative. J Atr Fibrillation 2017;10(4):1655.

23. Hanke T. Surgical management of the left atrial appendage: a must or a myth? Eur J Cardiothorac Surg 2018;53(suppl_1):i33–8.

Left Atrial Appendage Closure

Technical Considerations of Endocardial Closure

Carlos E. Sanchez, MD[a],*, Steven J. Yakubov, MD[b], Anish Amin, MD[b], Arash Arshi, MD[b]

KEYWORDS

- Nonvalvular atrial fibrillation • Left atrial appendage • Left atrial appendage closure
- Oral anticoagulant • Transesophageal echocardiography • Computed tomography angiography

KEY POINTS

- Left atrial appendage (LAA) closure has emerged as a safe and effective therapy for the prevention of stroke in patients with atrial fibrillation.
- Understanding the LAA anatomy, including morphology and dimensions, is essential for preprocedure planning, size selection, avoidance of complications, and successful device deployment.
- Transesophageal echocardiography (TEE) and computed tomography angiography (CTA) are the most frequent imaging modalities used to evaluate the LAA.
- TEE is the preferred mode to evaluate the LAA anatomy and rule out thrombi, but CTA provides the most comprehensive images of the LAA and surrounding structures.
- Upcoming LAA closure technologies focus on precise positioning and repositioning to reduce complication rates.

 Video content accompanies this article at http://www.cardiacep.theclinics.com.

INTRODUCTION

Atrial fibrillation is the most common clinically encountered arrhythmia.[1] The primary goal of therapy is to reduce rates of stroke and thromboembolism, and atrial fibrillation is ideally treated with oral anticoagulant therapy (OAC).[2] However, long-term compliance remains a significant issue and some patients are not candidates for anticoagulation. Left atrial appendage closure (LAAC) has been shown to be an effective method for reduction of cardioembolic stroke risk in patients who are not candidates for long-term anticoagulation.[3–5] An endocardial LAAC implant, although

intuitive, requires a sound understanding of left atrial and left atrial appendage (LAA) anatomy. Multimodality imaging can facilitate implant success and efficiency while reducing the risk of complications.

The LAA is an embryonic blind pouch located anterolaterally in the atrioventricular groove of the heart. The LAA can be divided into 2 distinct regions: (1) the nonfunctional LAA, generally recognized as the ostium and the landing zone of LAAC devices, is histologically derived from the pulmonary veins and morphologically visualized as a smooth walled structure; (2) the functional LAA is histologically derived from the left atrium

[a] Advanced Structural Heart Disease, OhioHealth Riverside Methodist Hospital, 3705 Olentangy River Road Suite 100, Columbus, OH 43214, USA; [b] OhioHealth Riverside Methodist Hospital, 3705 Olentangy River Road Suite 100, Columbus, OH 43214, USA
* Corresponding author.
E-mail address: Carlos.Sanchez@ohiohealth.com

Card Electrophysiol Clin 12 (2020) 47–54
https://doi.org/10.1016/j.ccep.2019.11.002

and is characterized by a pectinated appearance.[6] Within this context the LAA has a variable morphology and position. There are several anatomic relationships of importance, including the superior orientation of the pulmonary artery, posterior orientation of the left superior pulmonary vein, and the inferiorly directed mitral annular apparatus inclusive of the circumflex artery and great cardiac vein. Other significant structures include the overlying phrenic nerve, which is often laterally positioned, and the superiorly oriented subendocardial fibers of the Bachman bundle. Appropriate delivery of an LAAC device excludes the functional portion of the LAA, eliminating the site of largest thrombus formation, without affecting important surrounding structures.

LEFT ATRIAL APPENDAGE CLOSURE
Preprocedural Imaging

Typically, the LAA has multiple lobes with wide anatomic variations in its length, ostium size, and shape. The endocardial surface of the LAA has multiple pectinate muscles creating a trabecular structure. These anatomic characteristics, combined with slow blood flow creating stagnation commonly found in the LAA of patients with atrial fibrillation, promote a favorable milieu for thrombus formation. The LAA is the source of more than 90% of all thrombi in patients with nonvalvular atrial fibrillation (NVAF),[7] hence the reason long-term anticoagulation is indicated.

Transcatheter devices to exclude the LAA have emerged over the last decade to reduce the risk of stroke in patients with NVAF and high bleeding risk from long-term anticoagulation. At present, there are several LAA occlusion devices available worldwide.[8] The WATCHMAN device (Boston Scientific, Natick, MA) is presently the only LAA occlusion device approved by the US Food and Drug Administration in the United States for patients with NVAF at high risk for stroke.

Transesophageal echocardiography (TEE) and computed tomography angiography (CTA) are the most frequent imaging modalities used to evaluate the LAA. At present, TEE is the preferred mode to evaluate the LAA anatomy and rule out thrombi, but CTA provides the most comprehensive images of the LAA and surrounding structures. CTA assessment of the LAA has consistently shown larger ostial measurements relative to transesophageal or intracardiac ultrasonography.[9] CTA can also be used to assist in ruling out LAA thrombus. Attention to the LAA imaging protocol by CTA is essential to improve the positive predictive value for LAA thrombus detection. Delaying imaging 30 to 60 seconds after contrast bolus injection during imaging acquisition is important to differentiate a true filling defect from incomplete contrast mixing with stagnant blood flow in the LAA. With delayed imaging, defects present in the LAA 60 seconds after contrast administration are more likely to represent thrombus.[10] In contrast, in patients without filling defects visible in the LAA, a negative predictive value greater than 96% has been reported. Therefore, additional TEE may not be necessary to rule out LAA thrombus in the absence of filling defects on CTA.[11]

Given the wide anatomic variations of the LAA, preprocedural imaging with CTA to define the anatomy and its implications on endocardial and epicardial exclusion is becoming increasingly important. A recent LAA morphologic nomenclature based on multiplanar reconstruction cardiac CTA has classified the LAA into 4 categories based on their distinct shapes: (1) windsock, with 1 long dominant lobe; (2) chicken wing, with 1 dominant lobe with prominent bend; (3) cauliflower, with short LAA with multiple small lobes; and (4) cactus with 1 dominant central lobe that branches out to secondary lobes[12] (**Fig. 1**). Multiplanar reconstruction CTA is also a valuable tool to define dimensions of specific LAA anatomic structures, including the number of lobes, depth of the LAA, and maximal ostium diameter, essential for device sizing. Detailed anatomic information of the LAA provides important information for operators to create an implanting strategy and avoid complications, especially in cases in which challenging LAA anatomy is encountered. Potential LAA anatomic variations that may exclude the use of specific closure devices or pose a higher risk for complications include a very large LAA (>40 mm) or very short depth and severe lobe angulation.

Venous Access

Femoral venous access is obtained using the modified Seldinger technique. Our preferred practice is to use ultrasonography guidance to visualize the femoral vein, and to access the vein with a micropuncture needle and sheath. A guidewire is inserted, and the tract is dilated. A suture-mediated closure system such as the Perclose ProGlide (Abbot Vascular) may be deployed at this point, followed by insertion of an 8-Fr sheath. If intracardiac echocardiography is planned, a second femoral venous access is obtained inferior to the initial access in a similar fashion.

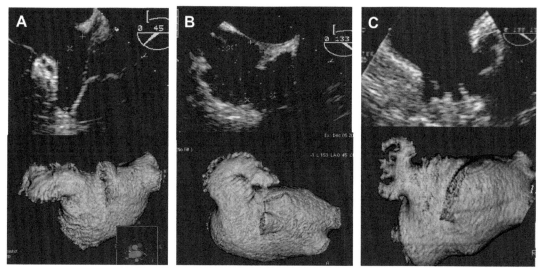

Fig. 1. LAA morphology showing (*A*) windsock with 1 dominant lobe; (*B*) chicken wing with sharp bend in the dominant lobe; (*C*) cauliflower with limited overall LAA length.

Transseptal Access

Optimal transseptal access location is an essential part of the procedure to facilitate LAAC. For most LAAC devices the ideal site of transseptal puncture is at the inferior and posterior aspect of the fossa ovalis. The puncture site location helps align the delivery sheath to the device-landing zone in the LAA, allowing optimal orientation and positioning of the device during deployment. The site of transseptal puncture is typically very precise, requiring optimal imaging. Because obtaining the precise location in the fossa may be challenging, echocardiographic (TEE or intracardiac echocardiography [ICE]) (**Fig. 2**) guidance is essential to improve safety and accuracy of the puncture site within the interatrial septum, although fluoroscopic imaging is often helpful for transseptal needle orientation.

Transesophageal echocardiographic guidance in conjunction with fluoroscopic imaging is traditionally used. The septum is crossed with a Swartz SL1 transseptal sheath (St. Jude Medical, Plymouth, MN) and NRG radiofrequency needle (NRG Transseptal Needle, Baylis Medical, Montreal, QC, Canada) via femoral vein access. Following transseptal puncture, a mean LAA pressure is often recorded. LAA dimensions should be assessed when the mean LAA pressure is greater than 12 mm Hg.[13] Anticoagulation with heparin is administered before transseptal puncture, and additional anticoagulation is given as needed to maintain activated clotting time (ACT) greater than 250 seconds. A 230-cm ProTrack pigtail guidewire (Baylis Medical Inc), chosen for its stiff proximal portion and large soft distal coil, is advanced and retained in left atrium under fluoroscopic guidance. For safety reasons,

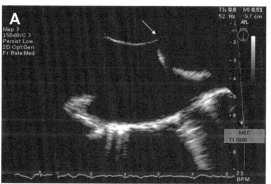
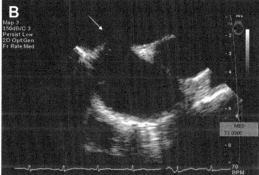

Fig. 2. Transseptal crossing under TEE guidance with bicaval (*A*) and short-axis (*B*) views to confirm inferoposterior needle location tenting the fossa ovalis (*arrow*).

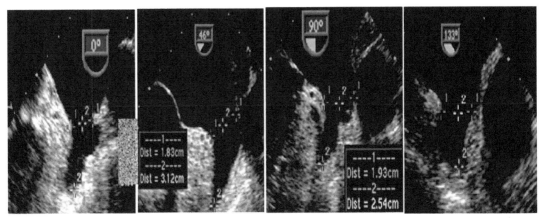

Fig. 3. Views of the LAA obtained in 0°, 45°, 90°, and 135° angulations for intraprocedural measurements.

these wires are preferred to stiff wires anchored in the pulmonary veins. The transseptal sheath is then removed carefully, maintaining wire access in the left atrium. After TEE or ICE characterization of the LAA anatomy and dimensions, and exclusion of thrombus, the 14-Fr LAAC access sheath is advanced to the left atrium over the stiff pigtail wire. The stiff wire is removed through a 6-Fr pigtail catheter placed in the LAAC access sheath. The pigtail catheter is gently advanced into the LAA. Right anterior oblique (RAO) cranial and RAO caudal cineangiography images of the LAA are obtained. The LAAC device is sized using all modalities (CTA, TEE or ICE, and angiography). The LAA device is delivered by the described technique for each specific device.

Procedural Anticoagulation

Anticoagulation with a 100-IU/kg bolus of heparin is recommended for a target ACT of 250 to 300 seconds. The entirety of the bolus may be given after venous access, or after transseptal access. In many practices, half the bolus (50 IU/kg) is administered after venous access is obtained, and an additional 50 IU/kg of heparin is given after successful transseptal puncture. Every 30 minutes, the ACT should be rechecked and additional heparin should be given to maintain the ACT between 250 and 300 seconds.

DEVICE DELIVERY, DEPLOYMENT, AND REPOSITIONING
Periprocedural Imaging

Successful device selection and implantation depends on obtaining accurate LAA dimensions. Although the shape of the LAA can influence the risk of stroke, LAAC depends less on LAA shape

and mostly on the ostial dimension and LAA length. Transesophageal echocardiography is the most common ultrasonography source for LAAC. Images of the LAA are obtained in 0°, 45°, 90°, and 135° angulations (**Fig. 3**). Three-dimensional TEE has been shown to more closely correlate to computed tomography–acquired measurements compared with two-dimensional echocardiography. Intraprocedural measurements using fluoroscopy or ultrasonography imaging should rely on the maximal dimensions obtained to avoid device undersizing.

The fluoroscopic working view for LAAC begins with an anteroposterior (AP) projection guiding access into the anterior lobe of the LAA with counterclockwise rotation of the pigtail catheter. The device delivery sheath is advanced to the ostium of the LAA using the pigtail as a rail. The working projection for device deployment remains the RAO 30°, CAU 20° projection, which correlates to the 135° TEE view. Correlation between angiographic projections and TEE angulations are described in **Table 1**.

The implant considerations for modern LAAC devices can be divided into those for nitinol cage–style devices and ball and disc–style

Table 1
Correlation between angiographic projections and transesophageal echocardiography angulations

Fluoroscopic Projection	TEE Angulation (°)
AP cranial	0
RAO 30°/CRA 20°	45
RAO 30°	90
RAO 30°/CAU 20°	135

Abbreviations: CAU, caudal; CRA, cranial.

devices. All devices are held in position through the radial forces across either the shoulders of a nitinol cage or the ball of a ball and disc device. Nitinol cage devices are ideally positioned with the shoulders of the device at or just distal to the LAA ostium, whereas ball and disc devices are positioned with the ball 1 cm distal to the LAA ostium at the ostium of the functional LAA. The landing zone is determined after careful evaluation of both the ultrasonography images and an LAA angiogram.

WATCHMAN DEPLOYMENT (BOSTON SCIENTIFIC)

WATCHMAN device selection is made to achieve a compression rate between 8% and 20%. The primary limitation of delivering nitinol cage devices from the perspective of sizing is obtaining enough LAA length to accommodate the maximal width of the device at the LAA ostium. Device anchoring occurs through radial tension applied across the shoulders of the device. Ideal positioning of the device places the shoulders at or just distal to the LAA ostium. Advancement of the WATCHMAN Deliver Sheath (WDS), most often the double curve sheath, into the LAA is guided by aligning the radiopaque maker band corresponding with the size of device chosen to the LAA ostium. The pigtail catheter can be withdrawn at this point, maintaining adequate WDS positioning because the sheath can advance forward during withdrawal of the pigtail. Similarly, counterclockwise rotation of the WDS may be required to maintain the appropriate angulation during withdrawal of the pigtail catheter and advancement of the WDS to the appropriate depth in the LAA. As the WATCHMAN device catheter is advanced within the WDS, the position of the feet of the device relative to the end of the delivery catheter should be assessed. As the tip of the delivery catheter aligns with the distal portion of the sheath, the sheath and catheter are locked together by moving the WDS proximally toward the WATCHMAN catheter. The WATCHMAN device is unsheathed with a left to right hand motion of the WDS. The WATCHMAN device catheter should always remain firmly fixed to limit forward movement. Deployment of larger devices, particularly the 30-mm and 33-mm devices, may require firm forward pressure to ensure that the device does not slip backward as the large shoulders are unsheathed.

Once the device is deployed the PASS criteria can be applied before releasing the WATCHMAN. The PASS criteria include an assessment of device position, anchoring, size, and seal. Device position is assessed to recognize that the functional LAA and all relevant pectinate muscles are excluded and the device has proper positioning and no deformation. Anchoring is assessed with a tug test to show that the device is unlikely to dislodge acutely. Size is measured through serial ultrasonography views to demonstrate 8% to 20% compression at the level of the shoulders. In addition, device seal is reviewed through color Doppler in serial views to ensure that no significant gaps are present. Angiography may be helpful in assessing proper positioning.

If a WATCHMAN device fulfills the PASS criteria it can be released. Should the device need to be repositioned, the device may be partially or fully recaptured. In the setting of device deployment that is considered too deep within the LAA, the device may be partially recaptured by holding the WATCHMAN device catheter firmly and advancing the WDS over the device shoulders. At this point the entire system may be withdrawn to the new landing position and deployed again. Should the initial device deployment be determined to be excessively proximal and the operator wishes to complete a deeper implantation, the device needs to be fully recaptured. The same steps are taken as a partial recapture, this time advancing the sheath over the shoulders and the feet. Often a fully recaptured device is considered to be unable to be redeployed because of deformation of the device itself or device catheter and a new device needs to be obtained.

LAAs with short working lengths or an inability to maintain access along the length of the LAA long axis can pose particular concerns for WATCHMAN delivery. In the case of short working length (see **Fig. 1**A), the LAA can be explored for lobes that allow more distal advancement of the WDS to gain more working length, or the device can be advanced just slightly as the feet exit the WDS and before the shoulders are unsheathed. Care should be taken in each of these scenarios to avoid mechanical complication of the LAA. For anatomies requiring excessive torque on the WDS, device delivery can result in a canted deployment and inadequate sealing. If the anterior lobe is predominant on CTA and/or TEE (which is the most common finding), this lobe is preferential for deployment for best alignment of the device with the LAA ostium. If excessive torque on the WDS is needed, the first consideration should be to change the WDS to a single curve or anterior curve sheath. The anterior curve is most useful for predominant anterior lobes of the LAA, when the double curve WDS fails. The single curve is most useful when the predominant lobe is posterior and the double curve WDS fails. Occasionally a different location with transseptal puncture can facilitate device delivery.

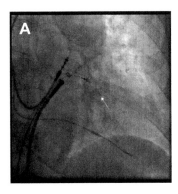
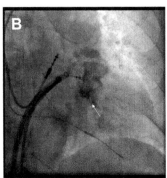

Fig. 4. Complete shoulder protrusion (*arrows*) without (*A*) and with contrast (*B*) of the device.

Short appendage lengths pose significant potential problems, especially those with angulated distal lobes (chicken wing anatomy) (see **Fig. 1**B). The preferred strategy is to avoid, if possible, deployment of the distal device past the angulation. The major risk is LAA perforation with straightening of the lobe. If the ostial width and LAA length are severely mismatched on pre-deployment imaging, it is usually best to avoid implantation of an endocardial device. This mismatch may also be seen with other anatomic variations. Ostial measurements greater than 32 mm, which are rare, often do not allow appropriate compression of available WATCHMAN devices, and these appendages should be avoided with WATCHMAN.

Device deformation may occur during deployment. The most common deformation involves an inability of the device to fully expand, which is visualized as excessive compression of the device, and is secondary to too distal deployment or an excessively small lobe, not allowing device expansion. Solutions involve a more proximal deployment or choosing another lobe for device deployment. This situation may also necessitate a delivery sheath change.

Although a common landmark for landing the device is the circumflex artery, often shoulder protrusion of the device into the left atrium can occur. If tug testing reveals a stable position, PASS criteria are fulfilled and no peridevice leak is seen, this position may be acceptable. Excessive shoulder protrusion usually necessitates recapturing and redeploying the device, or changing device size (**Fig. 4**, Video 1). Risk of late embolization is not acceptable.

Observation of pericardial effusion is rigorously monitored. This effusion is avoided by precise transseptal access and single deployment of the LAA occlusion device, with minimization of recapturing. Although TEE or ICE guidance is used, it may be difficult to fully evaluate effusions, especially in patients with previous cardiac surgeries.

Often transthoracic echocardiography can be helpful. Proficiency in pericardial drainage techniques with micropuncture technique is necessary. The ability to contain large effusions with autotransfusion or device deployment with additional closure devices (Amplatzer Vascular Plug II, atrial septal occluder devices) may be necessary. Surgical repair of large LAA ruptures may be necessary but is very uncommon.

WATCHMAN FLX (BOSTON SCIENTIFIC)

The WATCHMAN FLX received the Conformité Européene (CE) mark in 2019 with limited market release, and is under investigation in the United States. The WATCHMAN FLX offers several advantages compared with the WATCHMAN system (**Fig. 5**). The device has a soft, closed distal tip to minimize risk of LAA injury. Because of its shorter length, the device can be used in LAAs with functional depths as little as half the device diameter. The FLX system also has 18 struts and 2 rows of anchors to allow better conformation to asymmetric LAA anatomy with the potential for less peridevice leak. The threaded insert of the WATCHMAN FLX protrudes less than on the

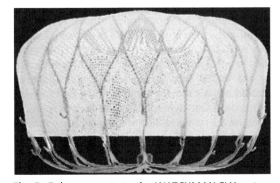

Fig. 5. Enhancements to the WATCHMAN FLX system include a shorter device length, closed atraumatic distal end, recessed threaded insert, additional struts, and longer polytetrafluoroethylene lining. (*Courtesy of* Boston Scientific, Natick, MA; with permission.)

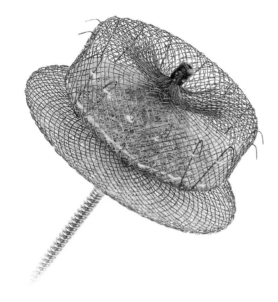

Fig. 6. The AMPLATZER Amulet consists of a nitinol frame covered by a polyester patch. The device has a distal lobe with stabilizing wires that help secure its position within the LAA neck, attached via a waist to a proximal disc that covers the ostium. (*Courtesy of* Abbott, Inc., Abbott Park, Il; with permission.)

WATCHMAN device, which may reduce the risk of device-related thrombus. The procedural technique is similar in principle to the WATCHMAN, with a few notable differences. The WATCHMAN FLX can be fully recaptured and redeployed without removal. The device can also be partially deployed so that it forms a ball, and the position can be adjusted proximally and distally. Because of its atraumatic tip, forward advancement of the device carries less risk of LAA injury.

AMPLATZER AMULET (ABBOTT)

The AMPLATZER Amulet LAAC Device received the CE mark in 2013, and is an investigational device in the United States. The AMPLATZER Amulet device is designed with a distal lobe that is deployed within the LAA and a proximal disc that is seated on the LA side of the LAA ostium, thereby sealing the LAA (**Fig. 6**). The device requires a functional LAA depth of only 12 mm, and may be suitable for small LAAs. Sizing is based on multimodal imaging, and CTA, fluoroscopy, and transesophageal or intracardiac echocardiographic methods are all acceptable. Device sizing is based on the maximal dimension of the landing zone. Maximum LAA neck diameter is recorded, and the device is typically oversized 2 to 4 mm. For more oval landing zones, less oversizing is recommended.

Access to the LAA is essentially the same as for the WATCHMAN device. Deployment of the AMPLATZER Amulet device is completed through an inferior transseptal puncture, after which a marker pigtail is advanced into the LAA. The AMPLATZER TorqVue Delivery Sheath is advanced into the LAA and the pigtail is removed from the sheath. Identification of the LAA ostium is critical to accurate placement of the device, and this is typically achieved in the RAO-cranial projection. The sheath should be advanced to the landing zone, approximately 12 to 15 mm distal to the LAA ostium. When advancing the Amulet device through the delivery sheath, as the device crosses the septum the system may slightly straighten. Gentle forward tension may need to be applied to the sheath to avoid losing position. The device is advanced to the tip of the sheath, and the sheath is retracted until the ball of the distal lobe of the Amulet is formed. The position of the Amulet can then be fine-tuned by advancement or retraction of the system. Counterclockwise torque may need to be applied to align the device coaxial to the LAA orifice. When a satisfactory position is achieved, the lobe is fully deployed by advancement of the delivery cable. The disc is deployed by advancing the cable and simultaneously retracting the sheath. The device may be gently tugged while observing on fluoroscopy and echocardiography to verify stability. There are 5 additional criteria that must be fulfilled to ensure device stability. (1) There must be some compression of the device. (2) There should be a visible waist to the device with separation of the lobe and disc. (3) The device should be oriented perpendicularly to the LAA neck. (4) The disc should be concave, which confirms appropriate tension on the device. (5) Two-thirds of the Amulet lobe should be distal to the circumflex artery on echocardiography. After these criteria are confirmed, the device can be released by counterclockwise rotation of the delivery cable. If the device position or stability is unsatisfactory, the Amulet can be fully recaptured and repositioned. Positioning of the device can be established through standard ultrasonography and fluoroscopic imaging with careful attention paid to the mitral valve and left superior pulmonary vein to assess for impingement of these structures by the disc.

VENOUS ACCESS SITE CLOSURE

After removal of the femoral venous sheath, closure may be performed by completing the previously deployed Perclose. This technique is preferred for reliability of closure and to assist in early ambulation. In cases in which preclosing was not performed, alternatives include manual compression or use of a figure-of-eight stitch.

DISCLOSURE STATEMENT

Dr C.E. Sanchez: consulting for Boston Scientific. Dr S.J. Yakubov: medical advisory board for Boston Scientific. Dr A. Amin: medical advisory board for Boston Scientific. Dr A. Arshi: no disclosures.

SUPPLEMENTARY DATA

Supplementary data related to this article can be found online at https://doi.org/10.1016/j.ccep. 2019.11.002.

REFERENCES

1. Wolf PA, Abbott RD, Kannel WB. Atrial fibrillation as an independent risk factor for stroke: the Framingham study. Stroke 1991;22:983–8.

2. January CT, Wann LS, Alpert JS, et al. 2014 AHA/ACC/HRS guideline for the management of patients with atrial fibrillation: a report of the American College of Cardiology/American Heart Association task force on practice guidelines and the Heart Rhythm Society. J Am Coll Cardiol 2014;64:e1–76.

3. Holmes DR, Reddy VY, Turi ZG, et al, Protect AF Investigators. Percutaneous closure of the left atrial appendage versus Warfarin therapy for prevention of stroke in patients with atrial fibrillation: a randomized non-inferiority trial. Lancet 2009;374:534–42.

4. Holmes DR, Kar S, Price MJ, et al. Prospective randomized evaluation of the Watchman left atrial appendage closure device in patients with atrial fibrillation versus long-term Warfarin therapy: the PREVAIL trial. J Am Coll Cardiol 2014;64:1–12.

5. Beigel R, Wunderlich NC, Yen Ho S, et al. The left atrial appendage: anatomy, function and non-invasive evaluation. JACC Cardiovasc Imaging 2014;7:1251–65.

6. Moorman A, Webb S, Brown Nigel A, et al. Development of the heart: (1) formation of the cardiac chambers and arterial trunks. Heart 2003;89(7):806–14.

7. Blackshear JL, Odell JA. Appendage obliteration to reduce stroke in cardiac surgical patients with atrial fibrillation. Ann Thorac Surg 1996;61:755–9.

8. Asmarats L, Rodes-Cabau J. Percutaneous left atrial appendage closure: current device and clinical outcomes. Circ Cardiovasc Interv 2017;10:e005359.

9. Chow DH, Bieliauskas G, Sawaya FJ, et al. A comparative study of different imaging modalities for successful percutaneous left atrial appendage closure. Open Heart 2017;4:e000627.

10. Saw J, Lopes JP, Reisman M, et al. Cardiac computed tomography angiography for left atrial appendage closure. Can J Cardiol 2016;32:1033. e1–9.

11. Romero J, Husain SA, Kelesidis I, et al. Detection of left atrial appendage thrombus by cardiac computed tomography in patients with atrial fibrillation. Circ Cardiovasc Imaging 2013;6:185–94.

12. Wang Y, Di Biase L, Horton RP, et al. Left atrial appendage studied by computed tomography to help planning for appendage closure device placement. J Cardiovasc Electrophysiol 2010;21:973–82.

13. Tzikas A, Gafoor S, Meerkin D, et al. Left atrial appendage occlusion with AMPLATZER Amulet device: an expert consensus step-by-step approach. EuroIntervention 2016;11:1512–21.

Periprocedural Imaging for Left Atrial Appendage Closure

Computed Tomography, Transesophageal Echocardiography, and Intracardiac Echocardiography

Thomas S. Gilhofer, MD[a], Jacqueline Saw, MD, FRCPC, FSCAI, FSCCT[b],*

KEYWORDS

• Intracardiac echocardiography • Left atrial appendage closure • Periprocedural imaging
• Transesophageal echocardiography guiding

KEY POINTS

• Transesophageal echocardiography (TEE) allows real-time morphologic and functional assessment of the LAA and is the reference standard for thrombus detection pre-LAAC, for procedural guidance, and evaluation for peridevice leaks and device-related thrombus post-LAAC. 3D TEE is valuable in the differentiation between thrombus and pectinate muscle, and better correlation of measurements compared with computed tomography angiography (CTA).
• Intracardiac echocardiography (ICE) is increasingly used as an imaging alternative for procedural guidance during LAAC, especially in patients at high-risk for endotracheal intubation or contraindications to TEE.
• CTA is routinely performed in many centers for LAAC preplanning because of its superior spatial resolution and ability to depict the 3D relationship of the LAA and surrounding structures. It is also noninvasive, and does not cause esophageal discomfort or risk compared with TEE. It is used as an alternative to TEE for baseline imaging and post-LAAC device surveillance.

Percutaneous left atrial appendage closure (LAAC) is increasingly performed for stroke prevention for patients with nonvalvular atrial fibrillation (AF) with contraindications to oral anticoagulation (OAC). More than 90% of thrombi reside in the LAA[1] with nonvalvular AF, a trabeculated blind pouch with complex and highly variable anatomy. The two most commonly used devices for LAAC are WATCHMAN (Boston Scientific, Natick, MA) and Amplatzer Cardiac Plug (ACP)/Amulet (Abbott Vascular, Minneapolis, MN) devices. The success and complication rates with LAAC have dramatically improved with maturing experience, growing procedural familiarity, and preprocedural planning. Use of multimodality imaging including cardiac computer tomography angiography (CCTA), transesophageal echocardiography (TEE), or intracardiac echocardiography (ICE) in conjunction with fluoroscopy is critical for procedural safety and implant success. The main tasks for periprocedural imaging are to provide high-quality images of the LAA and its surrounding structures to:

[a] Interventional Cardiology, Division of Cardiology, Vancouver General Hospital, University of British Columbia, Vancouver, British Columbia, Canada; [b] Interventional Cardiology, Division of Cardiology, Vancouver General Hospital, University of British Columbia, 2775 Laurel Street, Level 9, Vancouver, British Columbia V5Z1M9, Canada
* Corresponding author.
E-mail address: jsaw@mail.ubc.ca

Card Electrophysiol Clin 12 (2020) 55–65
https://doi.org/10.1016/j.ccep.2019.11.007
1877-9182/20/© 2019 Elsevier Inc. All rights reserved.

- Rule out preexisting thrombus
- Provide adequate LAA measurements for device-sizing
- Guide placement of the delivery sheath
- Optimize positioning and guide deployment of the device
- Visualize peridevice leaks and uncovered proximal lobes
- Assess device stability to minimize the risk of embolization
- Evaluate for procedural complications, such as pericardial effusion and impingement of surrounding structures
- Diagnose or exclude device-related thrombus

Operators should become familiar with these imaging modalities for periprocedural imaging.

TRANSTHORACIC ECHOCARDIOGRAPHY

Baseline transthoracic echocardiography is mandatory to evaluate left atrium (LA) dimensions, volumes, and left ventricular (LV) function for patients for LAAC.[2,3] TEE can exclude contraindications for LAAC, such as valvular AF (severe mitral stenosis), other significant valve disease requiring surgery, a mechanical heart valve, or an LV thrombus requiring OAC. Transthoracic echocardiography is also commonly performed predischarge to rule out pericardial effusion and device embolization.[1]

TRANSESOPHAGEAL ECHOCARDIOGRAPHY

LAAC imaging requires an experienced echocardiographer with attention to detail and thorough knowledge of all the procedural steps and their sequence. TEE visualizes LAA morphology and flow patterns, and is currently the most widely accepted imaging tool for LAAC. It has high sensitivity and specificity (92% and 98%, respectively) for detecting LAA thrombi and high negative and positive predictive values (100% and 86%, respectively).[4–6] Besides a detailed anatomic and functional assessment of the LAA, preprocedural

planning also involves evaluation of accompanying structures, such as LA, LV, left upper pulmonary vein (LUPV), and mitral valve, and their relationship to each other.[4,7,8]

Detection of Left Atrial Appendage Thrombus

It is controversial whether sludge or dense spontaneous echo contrast (SEC) within the LAA should be regarded and therefore managed equivalently as organized thrombus.[9] However, the annual stroke rate with dense SEC within the LAA was reported to be 18.2% without OAC and 4.5% on adjusted-dose warfarin. The presence of an LAA thrombus was shown to triple the overall stroke rate.[10] Thrombi in LAA and LA need to be excluded before safely proceeding with any invasive procedure involving the left-sided heart chambers. LAA thrombi are easily missed because of the complex three-dimensional (3D) anatomic features of the LAA and of the thrombus itself. Artifacts caused by acoustic shadowing from the pulmonary vein (PV) ridge or valve prostheses can overdiagnose thrombi. Pectinate muscles can also be misinterpreted as thrombi[4] but X-plane views can help with differentiation. Ultrasound contrast agents are helpful in evaluating subtle filling defects (**Fig. 1**).[11]

Three-Dimensional Transesophageal Echocardiography

3D TEE has become widely available in recent years. Technical advancements including software upgrades and higher resolution probes have substantially improved imaging support of complex interventional procedures, such as LAAC, with more reliable measurements compared with two-dimensional (2D), and better orientation in relationship to neighboring structures. 3D TEE measurements better correlate with multidetector computer tomography.[12–14] LAA volume calculations and volume-derived ejection fraction can only be obtained by 3D TEE.[15,16] It helps additionally in the differentiation

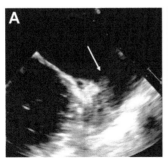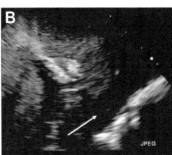

Fig. 1. (*A*) Two-dimensional TEE showing spontaneous echocardiographic contrast (*arrow*) in the LAA. (*B*) Two-dimensional TEE with use of ultrasound contrast revealing filling defect of thrombus in the distal portion of LAA (*arrow*).

between thrombus and pectinate muscle.[7,15] 3D TEE is superior to 2D TEE for assessment of thrombus mobility; delineation of changes in thrombus structure, such as calcification, degeneration, or lysis; and findings are more reproducibly confirmed by a better interobserver agreement.[4,15] Furthermore, the potential of having 2D biplane imaging is valuable for difficult LAA angles. Prolonged use of 3D or 2D biplane modes should be avoided because it can cause overheating of the TEE imaging head in the esophagus, causing edema and deterioration of image quality. This risk is addressed by turning down the power output settings.[1]

Left Atrial Appendage Contractility

Functional assessment of the LAA can help with risk stratification of thromboembolism. During sinus rhythm the LAA is a contractile muscular sac with pulsatile blood flow and low risk of stasis and thrombosis, but with AF this pulsatile flow is replaced by a chaotic flow pattern of varying velocities.[4,17] Pulsed-wave Doppler measures the maximal flow velocity in the proximal third of the LAA.[18] Adequate flow velocities greater than 40 cm/s is correlated with low-risk of thrombus formation,[4] whereas velocities less than 40 cm/s were associated with higher stroke risk and presence of SEC,[19] and velocities less than 20 cm/s were associated with LAA thrombus and a higher incidence of thromboembolic events.[10,20,21] Careful evaluation of the LAA is therefore mandatory in case of velocities less than 40 cm/s before cardioversion or device intervention involving the LA and LAA.[4,21,22] Microbubble contrast agent is useful to better assess flow velocity within the LAA when Doppler signals are suboptimal.[4] Evaluation of blood flow or presence of thrombus within the LAA using color Doppler is optimized by setting the Nyquist limit low ($\leq$50 cm/s). E/é and é-velocity were also found to be independently associated with LAA thrombus,[23] supporting the hypothesis that elevated filling pressures in diastolic dysfunction contribute to stasis and thrombus formation.[4,24] Similarly, compromised LAA contractility on speckle-tracking and strain-based imaging also correlated to higher incidence of LAA clot formation.[4,25]

Procedural Transesophageal Echocardiography Guidance

A quick overview of the overall LV function, relevant valvular pathologies, and assessment of the pericardial space is recommended. Before proceeding with device implantation the operator needs to have adequate information on the anatomy of the LAA (size, depth, shape, additional lobes, complex pectination, and proximal septae) and surrounding structures. Because of its anterolateral location the LAA is the furthest cardiac structure from the TEE probe and optimal positioning of the probe is necessary to provide the best view of the long axis of the LAA. This is usually achieved with the probe positioned in the midesophagus and slightly retroflexed in a 50° to 70° plane. In this view, the LAA is seen in its longest depth with the mitral anulus and the circumflex artery located medially, and the PV ridge and LUPV located laterally to the LAA.[1] In case of a more anteriorly located LAA the long-axis is better viewed in a 0° to 50° plane, whereas a 70° to 90° plane is ideal for more laterally located LAA. The short-axis of the LAA is best viewed in a 135° plane, which visualizes the anterior and posterior aspect of the LAA. Because this imaging plane is technically challenging, a biplane mode at 45° may be helpful. Because of the frequent elliptical shape of the LAA this view commonly represents the widest dimension and therefore dictates the size of the device. In postprocedural follow-up most peridevice leaks (PDL) are found along the posterior portion of the LAA orifice (>90%).[1,26]

Device Sizing

For ACP/Amulet, the landing zone determines the size and position of the device and is measured at 10 mm inside the echocardiographic orifice (line connecting circumflex artery and PV ridge) for ACP or 12 mm for Amulet. For WATCHMAN, the anatomic orifice (line from circumflex artery inferiorly to a point 1–2 cm inside the tip of the PV ridge superiorly) is measured. To determine the widest dimensions, measurements in four different views (0°, 45°, 90°, and 135°) are obtained (**Fig. 2**).[1] Device sizing is typically upsized by 3 to 5 mm for ACP, 2 to 4 mm for Amulet, and by 9% to 25% for WATCHMAN.[27] LAA depth also needs to be taken into consideration to ensure that there is enough depth to accommodate the delivery system, which is especially important with the WATCHMAN device. The ACP/Amulet device is less reliant on depth for implantation.

Transseptal Puncture

Because of the anterolateral orientation of the LAA, a posterior and inferior puncture within the fossa ovalis is aimed to allow coaxial sheath alignment of the delivery system.[1]

The bicaval view is usually achieved with a 90° to 100° imaging plane and provides a craniocaudal

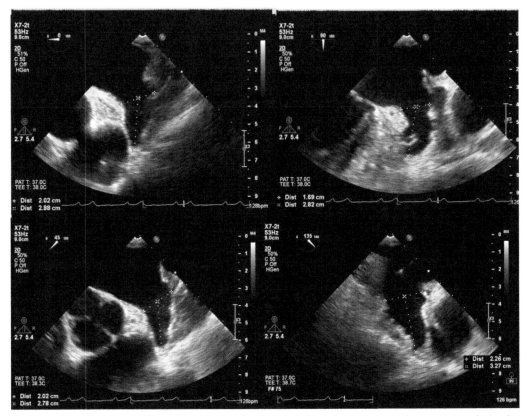

Fig. 2. Measurements of the LAA ostia and depth taken on 2D TEE for the parachute-shaped LAA occluder device in 0°, 45°, 90°, and 135° views.

or superoinferior view of the septum.[1] The interatrial septum (IAS) should be evaluated for its thickness, the presence of concomitant atrial septal aneurysm, patent foramen ovale, or atrial septal defects to help with selection of transseptal sheath and needle. Sometimes larger curves on the standard BRK1-XS (Abbott Vascular, Santa Clara, CA) or on the NRG radiofrequency (Bayliss Medical Mississauga, Canada) transseptal needles need to be created to reach the IAS, especially in case of atrial chamber enlargement. The radiofrequency needle is safer in very thick but also aneurysmatic membranes because less push is required and therefore the risk of perforation reduced. Once the transseptal needle is seen tenting the fossa ovalis in a mid-low position, the TEE angle is switched to 45° (short-axis) to view the anteroposterior orientation in relationship to the aortic valve. Switching back and forth between these two views or using biplane is often necessary to confirm an inferoposterior puncture. It is not recommended to go through a patent foramen ovale for LAAC because a coaxial placement of the delivery system is impossible, because of bias of the sheath anteriorly through the patent foramen ovale.[1]

Device Positioning

After successful transseptal puncture, the wire and the delivery catheter are advanced into the LUPV for exchanges. This is best achieved using a 45° view but with rotation of the imaging probe in a counterclockwise direction to shift the image from the septum to the LUPV.[1]

From the LUPV, a pigtail within the delivery system is guided into the LAA using the long-axis view (50°–90°). The optimal sheath position is coaxial with the long-axis and most anterior within the LAA, which is confirmed by the 45° to 60° and 135° views.[1] WATCHMAN needs the delivery system to be placed deep within the LAA, whereas the ACP/Amulet only requires coaxial position proximally at the landing zone. A final remeasurement of the LAA dimensions should be performed after confirming adequate volume loading to achieve LA pressure greater than 12 mm Hg, because volume status can significantly increase LAA orifice width and depth, potentially altering size selection.[28]

Device Position and Stability

Before device release, the degree of compression and the presence of PDL should be assessed. PDL appear as aliasing of color Doppler signal (Nyquist limit ≤ 50 cm/s[27]) at the gap between device and LAA wall for leaks less than 5 mm, and usually free-flow without aliasing in the presence of leaks greater than or equal to 5 mm.[1] If the position of the device is not satisfactory, the WATCHMAN and the ACP/Amulet devices are partially or fully recaptured and repositioned. Once a satisfying device position is achieved, stability of the WATCHMAN is tested by performing multiple gentle tugs with the cable, and by gentle constant traction of the disk with the ACP/Amulet device. The PASS criteria and five-signs of these devices should be achieved.

In a final assessment after release, the position of device, presence of any PDL, and pericardial effusion is reassessed. The IAS should be assessed using color Doppler to provide a landmark for future evaluation of the defect. Finally the pericardial space needs to be reassessed and compared with preimplantation images to detect potential pericardial effusion.

INTRACARDIAC ECHOCARDIOGRAPHY

ICE is an increasingly used alternative for procedural guidance, especially useful for patients with contraindications to TEE (eg, esophageal webs, varices, strictures/stenoses) or high-risk for endotracheal intubation. LAAC is safely performed under local anesthesia using ICE.[29,30] It can provide multiple views to detect LAA thrombi and help guide transseptal puncture and device implantation.[4,31,32] However, it is more invasive than TEE (requiring transvenous access), has more equipment cost, and has lower sensitivity for thrombus detection compared with TEE.[33] There is a significant learning curve with this technique, and there is heavy reliance on LAA measurements done on preprocedural TEE and CCTA for device sizing. There is also a need to have adjunctive imaging from procedural fluoroscopy for assessment of device position and PDL with ICE.[34] However, shorter procedural time caused by the lack of general anesthesia and not requiring an anesthesiologist or echocardiographer are significant advantages of ICE.[29,30,35]

Equipment

The two most widely used ICE-catheters are the ViewFlex Xtra (Abbot Vascular, Santa Clara, CA) and AcuNav (Biosense Webster, Irvine, CA). The ViewFlex is a 9F catheter, whereas the AcuNav is available in 8F and 10F catheter. Both have a working length of 90 cm and their shafts are deflected in four directions (anterior-posterior, right-left) with a maximum deflection angle of

120° with ViewFlex Xtra and 160° with AcuNav. At the tip of each catheter is an ultrasound transducer with 64-phased-array elements.[36] The ViewFlex Xtra probe is compatible with Philips and Zonare consoles. The AcuNav is compatible with Siemens and General Electric consoles.

Procedural Intracardiac Echocardiography Guidance

Views with intracardiac echocardiography

The ICE catheter is first inserted into the right atrium (RA) in a neutral position to image the long axis of the RA, tricuspid valve, and right ventricle (called home view). By rotating the ICE catheter clockwise, the long axis of the aortic valve, aortic root, LV outflow, pulmonary valve, and parts of the LA are visualized.[1] Further clockwise rotation allows visualization of the fossa ovalis. Gentle back and forth movements and tilting the catheter back and toward the right help to center the structure. The depth of field is adjusted to obtain full view of the IAS for transseptal puncture. Subtle clockwise rotation of the ICE catheter from the septum view provides imaging of the mitral valve. By adjusting the anterior/posterior knob of the catheter the LAA is visualized. Multiple views might be necessary to adequately scan the LAA and rule out thrombus before transseptal puncture. Despite suboptimal visualization of the LAA from the RA, technical success rate of LAAC with RA-based ICE guidance was shown to be as high as 97.5% with experienced operators.[29,36] Other positions to visualize the LAA from the right-heart include placing the ICE-catheter in the coronary sinus, the para-coronary sinus view (counterclockwise catheter from home view, and then deflect the probe posteriorly with the tip of the probe just below the coronary sinus), and the pulmonary artery; but it is challenging to advance the probe into these positions.[1] Imaging the LAA with the ICE catheter in the LA provides much better images, but does require crossing the IAS with the ICE probe, either through the same or another transseptal puncture (**Fig. 3**). This allows imaging the LAA from the LA and LUPV.[37]

Transseptal puncture

The ICE probe is positioned with retroflex tilt to visualize the IAS for transseptal puncture, which provides a craniocaudal view of the fossa ovalis. When adequate tenting is achieved in the inferior portion of the fossa, the next step is to guide the transseptal apparatus in an anteroposterior direction. By rotating the ICE catheter in a more clockwise direction the posterior part of the fossa is visualized. This movement is followed by gently rotating the transseptal apparatus in the same

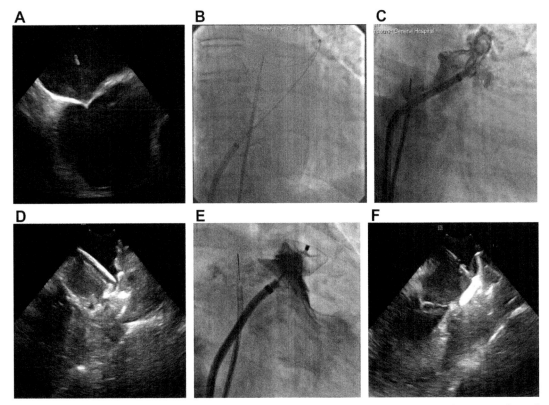

Fig. 3. ICE-guided LAAC with a lobe-and-disk device. (*A*) Transseptal puncture with precurved transseptal needle showing tenting of the fossa ovalis. (*B*) The ICE probe is advanced across the same transseptal puncture used for the device delivery sheath on fluoroscopy. (*C*) The ICE probe is slightly retroflex-tilted to visualize the LAA from the left atrium, and cineangiogram performed with the pigtail in the LAA. (*D*) ICE image showing the lobe of the device inside the LAA distal to the circumflex artery. (*E*) Fluoroscopy image showing the lobe and disk deployed. (*F*) ICE image showing the lobe and disk of the device in good position.

direction until adequate tenting in this inferior and posterior portion of the fossa is confirmed. Manipulation of the transseptal apparatus should be performed under ICE and fluoroscopic guidance.

Device deployment

Once the transseptal puncture is performed, the LAAC sheath is advanced back-and-forth across the IAS over a stiff Amplatz wire, to enlarge the puncture. We prefer to advance the ICE probe across this same transseptal puncture, by tilting and rotating the probe and sliding it through along the Amplatz wire. The ICE probe is then positioned facing the LAA, in a posterior-tilt position. Once the device is deployed within the LAA, the ICE probe is repositioned in the LUPV, or rotated inferiorly, to provide different angle imaging of the device within the LAA. Color Doppler is applied to assess for PDL. Position is also confirmed on fluoroscopy, and the remainder of the PASS and five-signs criteria assessed before release of device. At the end of the procedure, pericardial effusion is

assessed by advancing the ICE in the right ventricle.[1]

Three-dimensional intracardiac echocardiography

Currently, 3D ICE imaging is not widely available, with only one commercially available system, the ACUSON AcuNav V 3D Ultrasound Catheter (Siemens AG, Erlangen, Germany), which is only compatible with the Siemens ACUSON SC 2000 ultrasound system. Other devices will enter the market in the near future.

CARDIAC COMPUTER TOMOGRAPHY ANGIOGRAPHY

Multislice CCTA provides superior spatial resolution and 3D volumetric data to comprehensively assess the complex LAA anatomy and surrounding structures. Preprocedural imaging is a cornerstone of successful LAAC to rule out LAA thrombus in addition to optimally plan the procedure, guide device and equipment selection, and anticipate potential obstacles, which collectively can reduce procedural time, contrast dose, and complications. A small single-center study by Eng and coworkers (n = 24) showed that CCTA-guided LAAC was associated with improved device selection accuracy and procedural efficiency compared with 2D TEE, reducing procedural time and number of devices used.[38]

Left Atrial Appendage Thrombus Assessment

CCTA has a high sensitivity and negative predictive values of 96% to 100%[21,39–43] for detection of LAA thrombus, suggesting that patients without filling defects on CCTA do not need TEE. However, the positive predictive value is poor, because impaired contrast mixing can result in filling defects that can appear like LAA thrombus. A recent meta-analysis reported specificity of 41% to 92% and positive predictive value of only 41%.[9–12,44] Delayed imaging or use of dual-energy CT can help differentiate poor contrast filling from thrombus.[39,41,43,44] Dual-energy CCTA using rapid kilovoltage switching allows simultaneous acquisition of low- and high-tube-voltage data sets. This technique helps differentiate iodine-enhancing phenomena (eg, sluggish blood flow) from nonenhancing lesions (eg, thrombus) by means of the material decomposition method.[13,45] One study reported a positive predictive value of 100% with dual-energy source using cutoff values of 1.74 mg mL^{-1} iodine concentration for thrombus.[45] Delayed scans (imaging at least 30 seconds after contrast bolus) have become the standard for evaluation of LAA clot.[44,46] A filling defect caused by sluggish flow should improve on delayed imaging, whereas a filling defect persisting on delayed imaging is more likely to represent thrombus.[44,47] In a study of 55 patients with recent stroke, Hur and coworkers[45–48] reported a high concordance between CCTA (with late-phase imaging) and TEE for the detection of LAA thrombus, with overall sensitivity, specificity, and positive and negative predictive values of CCTA of 100%, 98%, 93%, and 100%, respectively. Another approach to improve contrast mixing in the LAA is to obtain delayed images in a prone position. Furthermore, thrombus mostly has an oval or round shape, whereas incomplete mixing appears more triangular-shaped with homogeneous signal intensity.[49]

Baseline Cardiac Computer Tomography Angiography Protocols

To properly assess LAA anatomy, advanced at least 64-detector scanners should be used. Our standard 320-detector scanner settings are as follows: rotation time 350 ms, collimation 320 × 0.5 mm, tube voltages 100 to 135 kV, and tube current 400 to 580 mA.[50] Contrast bolus of 50 to 90 mL is typically administered with flow-rate of 5 to 6 mL/s, followed by a mixture of 50% contrast/saline (20 mL) at the same rate, and a saline chaser (25 mL) at a rate of 3 mL/s. Automated peak enhancement detection in the LV is used for detection of the contrast bolus. After achieving +180 Hounsfield units (HU) craniocaudal scanning is initiated and images are acquired during an inspiratory breathhold of 8 to 10 seconds. Unlike coronary artery imaging, heart rate control is not mandatory because the intrinsic temporal resolution of 175 ms is acceptable for evaluation of the static LAA.[36,49] Electrocardiogram-gated tube current modulation enables radiation to be applied only during 30% to 40% of the R-R interval, which corresponds with late atrial diastole (phase of largest LA and LAA dimensions).[51] Because the LA is a highly compliant chamber, a volume bolus greater than 500 mL of saline should be administered before the scan, which is important for proper LAAC device sizing.[1]

Digital Post-processing

Various workstations are available for image processing enabling manipulation and reconstruction of the LAA and surrounding structures to guide LAAC: 3mensio (Pie Medical Imaging, Maastricht, The Netherlands), Aquarius Workstation (TeraRecon Inc, Foster City, CA), Brilliance Workspace (Philips Healthcare, Andover, MA), and Vitrea-Workststation (Vital, Toshiba Medical Systems Group Company). 3D digital reconstruction allows additional relational portrayal of conventional axial images. Multiplanar reconstruction creates volume images by stacking axial slices. Maximum-intensity projection is another volume-rendering technique that projects the voxel with the highest attenuation on every view. 3D volume-rendering offers the option to display the LAA from any desired perspective (**Fig. 4**), enabling selection of optimal correlative fluoroscopic angles during the procedure.

Device Selection

Careful assessment of shape and dimensions of the LAA are important before selecting the optimal device. Given the complex 3D LAA structure, standard axial views are inadequate for assessing the different dimensions of the LAA.[36] By using multiplanar reconstruction a view is identified where the LCX artery, the PV ridge, and the LAA ostium is clearly seen. For ACP/Amulet implantation the cross-section of the echocardiographic LAA

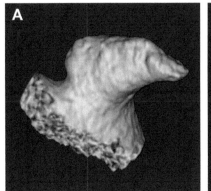
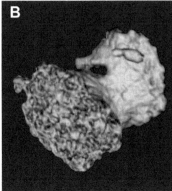
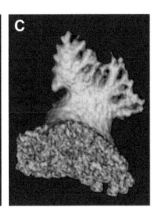

Fig. 4. 3D computed tomography angiography images showing the commonly classified shapes of LAA: (*A*) wind-sock, (*B*) chicken-wing, and (*C*) cactus.

ostium is obtained at right-angle projections to this plane to improve the coaxial measurement of the orifice. Then the widest diameter of the landing zone, 10 mm (for ACP) and approximately 12 mm (for Amulet) inside the orifice, is measured making sure that the measurement is coaxial. For WATCHMAN, the cross-section of the right angle projection to the anatomic LAA ostium is used for device sizing (**Fig. 5**). Suitable LAA diameters for device closures are: 12.6- to 28.5-mm landing zone for ACP, 12.6- to 32-mm landing zone for Amulet, and 17- to 31-mm anatomic ostium for WATCHMAN.[1] LAA orifices are frequently oval (>70% of cases), but can also be triangular, foot- or waterdrop-like, and round.[36,52] Marked sphericity at the site of the device implantation can pose additional challenges to the device selection. For the ACP/Amulet device, a depth of 10 to 15 mm measured from the LAA orifice to the back wall of the LAA is required. For the WATCHMAN, the depth is measured from the LAA ostium to the most distal tip of the distal lobe, which has to be as deep as the size of the device to be used. Therefore, preselecting the lobe of choice also facilitates selection of the appropriate access sheath (double-curve, single-curve, anterior curve) to achieve coaxial engagement into that lobe.[36]

Comparison of Cardiac Computer Tomography Angiography with Transesophageal Echocardiography

Most studies showed that 3D multiplanar CCTA provided the largest LAA measurements and can more accurately predict device size compared with 2D planar CT, TEE, and fluoroscopy.[53–55] 3D imaging with computed tomography angiography (CTA) or 3D TEE provide more accurate measurements of the LAA ostium and depth.[7] A small 28-patient study by Nakajima[8] demonstrated that measurement by 3D TEE yielded larger landing zone dimensions compared with 2D TEE. 3D TEE correlated better with CTA but was still undersized

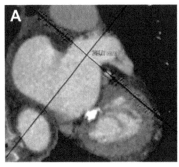
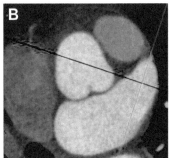
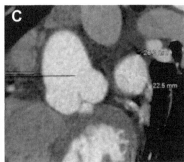

Fig. 5. Measurements of the LAA ostia for the parachute-shaped LAA occluder device on computed tomography angiography. (*A*) Cross-hair in an oblique multiplanar reconstruction view, positioned at the LAA ostia from the circumflex artery to a point 1–2 cm within the LUPV. (*B*) Ninety-degree oblique multiplanar reconstruction plane from (*A*), with cross-hair adjusted to be coaxial to the wall of the appendage. (*C*) Double-oblique planes adjusted from two prior views, to allow measurements of the LAA in the enface view.

(P = .022). Depth dimensions by 2D TEE were similarly smaller than 3D TEE, and both of which were smaller than CTA. Similar findings were reported by Saw[55] in a larger study (n = 50), where maximal LAA diameter was significantly larger for CTA (24.1 ± 4.7 mm) versus TEE (22.3 ± 4.9 mm) (P<.001). Wang[52] found that preprocedural CTA was associated with fewer device implantations per procedure and 100% success rate, at 1.2 devices/procedure in their study compared with 1.8 devices/procedure in the PROTECT-AF study.[5] The same group also found that CTA LAA sizing was consistently larger than 2D and 3D TEE (by 2–3 mm).[7]

Post-procedural Follow-up

CCTA is also a feasible alternative to TEE for device surveillance after LAAC to evaluate for position, embolization, device-related thrombus, residual contrast leak (patency), and pericardial effusion, avoiding the discomfort and risks associated with TEE.[27,56] An absence of contrast enhancement within the LAA without any PDL suggests complete neoendothelialization, whereas contrast enhancement in the LAA of less than 50 HU compared with the LA suggests incomplete neoendothelialization.[57,58] This represents a largely reviewer-independent method to interpret the images with regard to PDL. An association between a successfully occluded LAA and a linear attenuating coefficient of less than 100 HU in the LAA and an attenuation of less than 25% of the contrast opacification of the LA have also been described.[27] In the largest series comparing CCTA with TEE post-LAAC (n = 102), residual contrast patency in LAA is observed more frequently with CCTA (52%) compared with PDL on TEE (34.3%). Sealed appendages had greater device compressions compared with patent LAA.[56] However, the clinical significance of leaks observed on CCTA is unclear.

SUMMARY

Preprocedural imaging is instrumental for a successful LAAC procedure, encompassing detailed anatomic assessment of the LAA and surrounding structures, and accurate measurements for device sizing. These can facilitate device and equipment selection, shortens procedural duration, and enhances safety and outcomes with intraprocedural guidance with TEE or ICE.

DISCLOSURE

There was no funding or support for work performed for this article. Dr J. Saw has received unrestricted research grant supports from the Canadian Institutes of Health Research, Heart & Stroke Foundation of Canada, National Institutes of Health, AstraZeneca, Abbott Vascular, St. Jude Medical, Boston Scientific, and Servier; speaker honoraria from AstraZeneca, Abbott Vascular, Boston Scientific, and Bayer; consultancy and advisory board honoraria from AstraZeneca, Boston Scientific, and Abbott Vascular; and proctorship honoraria from Abbott Vascular and Boston Scientific.

REFERENCES

1. Saw J, Kar S, Price M. Left atrial appendage closure: mechanical approaches to stroke prevention in atrial fibrillation. Switzerland: Humana Press. Springer International Publishing AG; 2016.
2. Pritchett AM, Jacobsen SJ, Mahoney DW, et al. Left atrial volume as an index of left atrial size: a population-based study. J Am Coll Cardiol 2003; 41(6):1036–43.
3. Lang RM, Bierig M, Devereux RB, et al. Recommendations for chamber quantification: a report from the American Society of Echocardiography's Guidelines and Standards Committee and the Chamber Quantification Writing group, developed in conjunction with the European Association of Echocardiography, a branch of the European Society of Cardiology. J Am Soc Echocardiogr 2005;18(12):1440–63.
4. Beigel R, Wunderlich NC, Ho SY, et al. The left atrial appendage: anatomy, function, and noninvasive evaluation. JACC Cardiovasc Imaging 2014;7(12): 1251–65.
5. Acar J, Cormier B, Grimberg D, et al. Diagnosis of left atrial thrombi in mitral stenosis: usefulness of ultrasound techniques compared with other methods. Eur Heart J 1991;12(Suppl B):70–6.
6. Manning WJ, Weintraub RM, Waksmonski CA, et al. Accuracy of transesophageal echocardiography for identifying left atrial thrombi. A prospective, intraoperative study. Ann Intern Med 1995;123(11): 817–22.
7. Marek D, Vindis D, Kocianova E. Real time 3-dimensional transesophageal echocardiography is more specific than 2-dimensional TEE in the assessment of left atrial appendage thrombosis. Biomed Pap Med Fac Univ Palacky Olomouc Czech Repub 2013;157(1):22–6.
8. Nakajima H, Seo Y, Ishizu T, et al. Analysis of the left atrial appendage by three-dimensional transesophageal echocardiography. Am J Cardiol 2010; 106(6):885–92.
9. Hajjiri M, Bernstein S, Saric M, et al. Atrial fibrillation ablation in patients with known sludge in the left atrial appendage. J Interv Card Electrophysiol 2014;40(2):147–51.

10. Transesophageal echocardiographic correlates of thromboembolism in high-risk patients with nonvalvular atrial fibrillation. The Stroke Prevention in Atrial Fibrillation Investigators Committee on Echocardiography. Ann Intern Med 1998;128(8):639–47.

11. Yao SS, Ilercil A, Meisner JS, et al. Improved Doppler echocardiographic assessment of the left atrial appendage by peripheral vein injection of sonicated albumin microbubbles. Am Heart J 1997; 133(4):400–5.

12. Nucifora G, Faletra FF, Regoli F, et al. Evaluation of the left atrial appendage with real-time 3-dimensional transesophageal echocardiography: implications for catheter-based left atrial appendage closure. Circ Cardiovasc Imaging 2011;4(5):514–23.

13. Perk G, Biner S, Kronzon I, et al. Catheter-based left atrial appendage occlusion procedure: role of echocardiography. Eur Heart J Cardiovasc Imaging 2012;13(2):132–8.

14. Shah SJ, Bardo DM, Sugeng L, et al. Real-time three-dimensional transesophageal echocardiography of the left atrial appendage: initial experience in the clinical setting. J Am Soc Echocardiogr 2008;21(12):1362–8.

15. Anwar AM, Nosir YF, Ajam A, et al. Central role of real-time three-dimensional echocardiography in the assessment of intracardiac thrombi. Int J Cardiovasc Imaging 2010;26(5):519–26.

16. Chen OD, Wu WC, Jiang Y, et al. Assessment of the morphology and mechanical function of the left atrial appendage by real-time three-dimensional transesophageal echocardiography. Chin Med J (Engl) 2012;125(19):3416–20.

17. Li YH, Lai LP, Shyu KG, et al. Clinical implications of left atrial appendage function: its influence on thrombus formation. Int J Cardiol 1994;43(1):61–6.

18. Agmon Y, Khandheria BK, Gentile F, et al. Echocardiographic assessment of the left atrial appendage. J Am Coll Cardiol 1999;34(7):1867–77.

19. Fatkin D, Kelly RP, Feneley MP. Relations between left atrial appendage blood flow velocity, spontaneous echocardiographic contrast and thromboembolic risk in vivo. J Am Coll Cardiol 1994;23(4):961–9.

20. Li YH, Lai LP, Shyu KG, et al. Clinical implications of left atrial appendage flow patterns in nonrheumatic atrial fibrillation. Chest 1994;105(3):748–52.

21. Santiago D, Warshofsky M, Li Mandri G, et al. Left atrial appendage function and thrombus formation in atrial fibrillation-flutter: a transesophageal echocardiographic study. J Am Coll Cardiol 1994;24(1): 159–64.

22. Handke M, Harloff A, Hetzel A, et al. Left atrial appendage flow velocity as a quantitative surrogate parameter for thromboembolic risk: determinants and relationship to spontaneous echocontrast and thrombus formation. A transesophageal echocardiographic study in 500 patients with cerebral ischemia. J Am Soc Echocardiogr 2005;18(12): 1366–72.

23. Doukky R, Garcia-Sayan E, Gage H, et al. The value of diastolic function parameters in the prediction of left atrial appendage thrombus in patients with nonvalvular atrial fibrillation. Cardiovasc Ultrasound 2014;12:10.

24. Vigna C, Russo A, De Rito V, et al. Frequency of left atrial thrombi by transesophageal echocardiography in idiopathic and in ischemic dilated cardiomyopathy. Am J Cardiol 1992;70(18):1500–1.

25. Ono K, Iwama M, Kawasaki M, et al. Motion of left atrial appendage as a determinant of thrombus formation in patients with a low CHADS2 score receiving warfarin for persistent nonvalvular atrial fibrillation. Cardiovasc Ultrasound 2012;10:50.

26. Jaguszewski M, Manes C, Puippe G, et al. Cardiac CT and echocardiographic evaluation of peridevice flow after percutaneous left atrial appendage closure using the AMPLATZER cardiac plug device. Catheter Cardiovasc Interv 2015;85(2):306–12.

27. Saw J, Fahmy P, DeJong P, et al. Cardiac CT angiography for device surveillance after endovascular left atrial appendage closure. Eur Heart J Cardiovasc Imaging 2015;16(11):1198–206.

28. Spencer RJ, DeJong P, Fahmy P, et al. Changes in left atrial appendage dimensions following volume loading during percutaneous left atrial appendage closure. JACC Cardiovasc Interv 2015;8(15):1935–41.

29. Berti S, Paradossi U, Meucci F, et al. Periprocedural intracardiac echocardiography for left atrial appendage closure: a dual-center experience. JACC Cardiovasc Interv 2014;7(9):1036–44.

30. Fassini G, Dello Russo A, Conti S, et al. An alternative transseptal intracardiac echocardiography strategy to guide left atrial appendage closure: the first described case. J Cardiovasc Electrophysiol 2014;25(11):1269–71.

31. Blendea D, Heist EK, Danik SB, et al. Analysis of the left atrial appendage morphology by intracardiac echocardiography in patients with atrial fibrillation. J Interv Card Electrophysiol 2011;31(3):191–6.

32. Ren JF, Marchlinski FE, Supple GE, et al. Intracardiac echocardiographic diagnosis of thrombus formation in the left atrial appendage: a complementary role to transesophageal echocardiography. Echocardiography 2013;30(1):72–80.

33. Saksena S, Sra J, Jordaens L, et al. A prospective comparison of cardiac imaging using intracardiac echocardiography with transesophageal echocardiography in patients with atrial fibrillation: the intracardiac echocardiography guided cardioversion helps interventional procedures study. Circ Arrhythm Electrophysiol 2010;3(6):571–7.

34. Matsuo Y, Neuzil P, Petru J, et al. Left atrial appendage closure under intracardiac echocardiographic guidance: feasibility and comparison with

transesophageal echocardiography. J Am Heart Assoc 2016;5(10) [pii:e003695].

35. MacDonald ST, Newton JD, Ormerod OJ. Intracardiac echocardiography off piste? Closure of the left atrial appendage using ICE and local anesthesia. Catheter Cardiovasc Interv 2011;77(1):124–7.

36. Prakash R, Saw J. Imaging for percutaneous left atrial appendage closure. Catheter Cardiovasc Interv 2018;92(2):437–50.

37. Patti G, Mantione L, Goffredo C, et al. Intracardiac echocardiography with ultrasound probe placed in the upper left pulmonary vein to guide left atrial appendage closure: first description. Catheter Cardiovasc Interv 2019;93(1):169–73.

38. Eng MH, Wang DD, Greenbaum AB, et al. Prospective, randomized comparison of 3-dimensional computed tomography guidance versus TEE data for left atrial appendage occlusion (PRO3DLAAO). Catheter Cardiovasc Interv 2018;92(2):401–7.

39. Hong SJ, Kim JY, Kim JB, et al. Multidetector computed tomography may be an adequate screening test to reduce periprocedural stroke in atrial fibrillation ablation: a multicenter propensity-matched analysis. Heart Rhythm 2014;11(5):763–70.

40. Dorenkamp M, Sohns C, Vollmann D, et al. Detection of left atrial thrombus during routine diagnostic work-up prior to pulmonary vein isolation for atrial fibrillation: role of transesophageal echocardiography and multidetector computed tomography. Int J Cardiol 2013;163(1):26–33.

41. Martinez MW, Kirsch J, Williamson EE, et al. Utility of nongated multidetector computed tomography for detection of left atrial thrombus in patients undergoing catheter ablation of atrial fibrillation. JACC Cardiovasc Imaging 2009;2(1):69–76.

42. Patel A, Au E, Donegan K, et al. Multidetector row computed tomography for identification of left atrial appendage filling defects in patients undergoing pulmonary vein isolation for treatment of atrial fibrillation: comparison with transesophageal echocardiography. Heart Rhythm 2008;5(2):253–60.

43. Tang RB, Dong JZ, Zhang ZQ, et al. Comparison of contrast enhanced 64-slice computed tomography and transesophageal echocardiography in detection of left atrial thrombus in patients with atrial fibrillation. J Interv Card Electrophysiol 2008;22(3):199–203.

44. Romero J, Husain SA, Kelesidis I, et al. Detection of left atrial appendage thrombus by cardiac computed tomography in patients with atrial fibrillation: a meta-analysis. Circ Cardiovasc Imaging 2013;6(2):185–94.

45. Hur J, Kim YJ, Lee HJ, et al. Cardioembolic stroke: dual-energy cardiac CT for differentiation of left atrial appendage thrombus and circulatory stasis. Radiology 2012;263(3):688–95.

46. Hur J, Kim YJ, Lee HJ, et al. Dual-enhanced cardiac CT for detection of left atrial appendage thrombus in patients with stroke: a prospective comparison study with transesophageal echocardiography. Stroke 2011;42(9):2471–7.

47. Hur J, Kim YJ, Lee HJ, et al. Left atrial appendage thrombi in stroke patients: detection with two-phase cardiac CT angiography versus transesophageal echocardiography. Radiology 2009;251(3):683–90.

48. Romero J, Cao JJ, Garcia MJ, et al. Cardiac imaging for assessment of left atrial appendage stasis and thrombosis. Nat Rev Cardiol 2014;11(8):470–80.

49. Saw J, Lopes JP, Reisman M, et al. Cardiac computed tomography angiography for left atrial appendage closure. Can J Cardiol 2016;32(8):1033.e1-9.

50. van Rosendael PJ, Katsanos S, van den Brink OW, et al. Geometry of left atrial appendage assessed with multidetector-row computed tomography: implications for transcatheter closure devices. EuroIntervention 2014;10(3):364–71.

51. Patel AR, Fatemi O, Norton PT, et al. Cardiac cycle-dependent left atrial dynamics: implications for catheter ablation of atrial fibrillation. Heart rhythm 2008; 5(6):787–93.

52. Wang Y, Di Biase L, Horton RP, et al. Left atrial appendage studied by computed tomography to help planning for appendage closure device placement. J Cardiovasc Electrophysiol 2010;21(9):973–82.

53. Budge LP, Shaffer KM, Moorman JR, et al. Analysis of in vivo left atrial appendage morphology in patients with atrial fibrillation: a direct comparison of transesophageal echocardiography, planar cardiac CT, and segmented three-dimensional cardiac CT. J Interv Card Electrophysiol 2008;23(2):87–93.

54. Lopez-Minguez JR, Gonzalez-Fernandez R, Fernandez-Vegas C, et al. Comparison of imaging techniques to assess appendage anatomy and measurements for left atrial appendage closure device selection. J Invasive Cardiol 2014;26(9):462–7.

55. Saw J, Fahmy P, Spencer R, et al. Comparing measurements of CT angiography, TEE, and fluoroscopy of the left atrial appendage for percutaneous closure. J Cardiovasc Electrophysiol 2016;27(4):414–22.

56. Qamar SR, Jalal S, Nicolaou S, et al. Comparison of cardiac computerized tomography angiography and trans-esophageal echocardiography for device surveillance after left atrial appendage closure. EuroIntervention 2019;15(8):663–70.

57. Behnes M, Akin I, Sartorius B, et al. LAA occluder view for post-implantation evaluation (LOVE): standardized imaging proposal evaluating implanted left atrial appendage occlusion devices by cardiac computed tomography. BMC Med Imaging 2016;16:25.

58. Sawit ST, Garcia-Alvarez A, Suri B, et al. Usefulness of cardiac computed tomographic delayed contrast enhancement of the left atrial appendage before pulmonary vein ablation. Am J Cardiol 2012; 109(5):677–84.

Left Atrial Appendage Closure

Prevention and Management of Periprocedural and Postprocedural Complications

Ben Wilkins, MBChB, Motoki Fukutomi, MD, Ole De Backer, MD, PhD, Lars Søndergaard, MD, DMSc*

KEYWORDS

- Left atrial appendage closure • Complications • Prevention • Management

KEY POINTS

- The left atrial appendage closure procedure has important associated complications. Incidence, identification, avoidance, and management are discussed in this article.
- Complications can arise periprocedurally and include vascular access complications, transseptal puncture complications, pericardial effusion, device embolization, periprocedural stroke, and air embolus.
- Postprocedural complications include peridevice leak, device-related thrombus, and device erosion/late pericardial effusion.

INTRODUCTION

An appropriately cautious uptake of left atrial appendage closure (LAAC) has followed from early randomized trial evidence. In the PROTECT-AF[1] and PREVAIL[2] trials, LAAC was demonstrated to be noninferior to warfarin for the prevention of stroke in patients with nonvalvular atrial fibrillation (NVAF); however, a relatively high rate of procedural complications was feared to offset the perceived clinical benefit of the procedure. Minimizing the rate of periprocedural and postprocedural complications in LAAC is a critical aspect of improving patient outcomes and expanding this treatment option.

Potential complications in LAAC relate to 3 broad factors. First, the LAAC device itself, which comes with its limitations and for which correct device size selection and positioning is important.

Second, patient anatomy can vary widely and may cause challenges and demand high operator skills. Finally, the high incidence of comorbidities among patients undergoing LAAC means the procedure is frequently performed in a medically vulnerable patient population. Currently, percutaneous LAAC is mainly indicated for patients with NVAF and high bleeding risk during anticoagulant therapy.[3,4] Importantly, this patient cohort may tolerate procedural complications poorly, adding to the importance of mitigating procedural complications.

PERIPROCEDURAL COMPLICATIONS

Vascular Access

Vascular complications related to the femoral vein include puncture site bleeding, hematoma, arteriovenous fistula, pseudoaneurysm, deep vein

Department of Cardiology, Heart Center, Rigshospitalet, University of Copenhagen, Blegdamsvej 9, Copenhagen 2100, Denmark
* Corresponding author.
E-mail address: lars.soendergaard.01@regionh.dk

Card Electrophysiol Clin 12 (2020) 67–75
https://doi.org/10.1016/j.ccep.2019.10.003

thrombosis, and infection. In a metaanalysis of 1017 LAAC cases, access site complications occurred in 8.6% of the patients and were the most common adverse event.[5] However, ultrasound (US) -guided venous puncture is now frequently used and is associated with lower rates of both major and minor vascular complications as compared with palpation-guided puncture.[6,7] After the procedure, closure at the venous access is commonly done using a "figure-of-8" suture and direct compression. An alternative is the use of suture-based vascular closure devices (eg, Perclose ProGlide; Abbott Vascular, Santa Clara, CA, USA), which has been reported to significantly decrease the number of patients with prolonged bed rest and the frequency of hematoma when compared with manual compression alone.[8] Arterial puncture is not needed for LAAC procedures and should be avoided.

Transseptal Puncture Technique

A critical step in the LAAC procedure, cardiac tamponade and aortic perforation are identified as life-threatening complications of transseptal puncture. These serious complications can be virtually eliminated with the use of echocardiographic guidance with either transesophageal (TEE) or intracardiac echocardiography (ICE). For successful implantation of an LAAC device, the site of transseptal puncture is usually the inferoposterior part of the fossa ovalis. Anterior puncture of the fossa ovalis or crossing of a patent foramen ovale should be avoided, because this may compromise good maneuverability and coaxial alignment of the delivery sheath with the left atrial appendage (LAA).

Transseptal puncture may be challenging in case of thickened or aneurysmal interatrial septum. In such cases, the use of diathermy may allow septal crossing without additional forward pressure on the needle, thereby also preserving needle position on the septum. Balloon dilatation of the puncture site may also be necessary to allow safe passage of the LAAC delivery system if the septum is thickened or scarred.

Pericardial Effusion

Pericardial effusion and tamponade have been the main drivers of safety outcome data in the above-mentioned randomized LAAC trials. The PROTECT AF and PREVAIL trials reported a 4.2% and 1.9% rate of significant pericardial effusion requiring intervention, respectively. However, the rate of pericardial effusion has been reduced in more recent studies and registries to a range of less than 1% to 2%.[9–11]

The left atrial appendage is a thin-walled structure, which has epicardium at its outer surface across almost its entirety. Any instrumentation of the LAA by a delivery system and/or closure device can lead to pericardial bleeding owing to local trauma and the potential for cardiac tamponade. Adjacent structures, such as the pulmonary veins (PVs), may also be injured during the LAAC procedure and can also lead to pericardial effusion.

Because it is not uncommon for patients to have a small pericardial collection at baseline, this should be preoperatively evaluated with echocardiography to avoid confusion during interoperative or postprocedural checks. Following access to the left atrium, the use of a stiff guidewire to exchange to the delivery catheter is mandatory. The safest position of the stiff guidewire is in the left superior PV during advancement of the delivery system into the left atrium. Alternatively, a preshaped stiff guidewire (eg, Safari guidewire; Boston Scientific Inc, Boston, MA, USA) can be placed in the left atrium cavity as support when exchanging to the delivery system.

As a next step, careful navigation of the delivery system into the LAA is important. Several manufacturers provide a range of delivery system curvatures to accommodate the highly variable position of the LAA orifice and to maximize coaxial alignment with the LAA. The risk of trauma to the LAA can be reduced by advancing a pigtail catheter through the delivery system and into the LAA.[12] Subsequently, the LAA delivery catheter can be advanced over the pigtail into the LAA. Finally, the LAAC device should not be "pushed out" of the delivery catheter and is safer to be "unsheathed" at the initial phase. Interestingly, use of preprocedural cardiac computed-tomography (CT) planning has been shown to reduce the number of devices used per procedure, thereby theoretically reducing the risk for LAA trauma during device repositioning.[13]

Nearly 90% of pericardial effusions occur within 24 hours of the procedure.[14] Pericardial effusion can be managed conservatively, if limited. If the tear is located within the LAA, deployment of the closure device may potentially seal off the leak. Emergency placement of a percutaneous drain is necessary in case of hemodynamic instability and, occasionally, large-volume bleeding requiring pericardial aspiration with autotransfusion is required.[15] Rarely, bailout surgery with creation of a pericardial window or suturing of the LAA tear is required in case of failed pericardiocentesis or nonresolving pericardial bleeding.[16]

Device Embolization

Device embolization occurs in the setting of device malpositioning or inappropriate device sizing. Embolization is noted at 0.2% to 1% across a range of different LAAC devices.[9–11,17]

The most commonly available percutaneous LAAC devices are fixed to the LAA through physical compression of the device frame as well as small hooks or barblike projections that imbed in the LAA wall, giving early stability. Device undersizing can lead to insufficient radial force of the device and poor opposition of any stabilization hooks. On the other hand, device oversizing can cause excessive compression leading to physical expulsion from the LAA or important device deformation, which limits the ability of any tissue fixation hooks from engaging the LAA wall. Similarly, a device that is not coaxially aligned to the LAA or positioned too shallow may lose its mechanical performance and be prone to embolization.

Some LAA anatomies are associated with a higher risk of device embolization: a large diameter of the LAA landing zone leading to insufficient device compression, a wide-open tapering LAA ostium, limited LAA depth, or a more complex LAA morphology with, for example, multiple LAA lobes or a highly elliptical or angulated LAA.[17] An acutely angulated LAA implies that it is often not possible to completely oppose the fixation hooks from the LAAC device. Device-specific implantation strategies have been developed to mitigate embolic risk in such situations, including the "sandwich technique" for implantation of the AMPLATZER Amulet device (Abbott, Plymouth, MN, USA).[18] In all cases, a "tug-test" can be performed before device release to confirm a secure position within the LAA.

Generally, low embolization rates have been reported in the most recent LAAC studies and registries, which may be related to operator experience as well as better sizing of the LAA, for example, by use of cardiac CT scan.

Some device-specific criteria have been proposed to check before taking the final decision to release the LAAC device. For the WATCHMAN device (Boston Scientific Inc), the PASS criteria are commonly used[1,17]:

P	Position just distal to the LAA ostium
A	Anchoring is adequate with gentle "push-pull" test
S	Size of the device shows suitable compression of 8%–20%
S	Satisfactory Seal has been made with the LAA

Similarly, 5 prerelease ("CLOSE") criteria have been proposed to optimize deployment of the AMPLATZER Amulet device[19]:

C	Device lobe at least 2/3 distal to the Circumflex artery
L	Adequate Lobe compression
O	Perpendicular Orientation of the lobe within the LAA
S	Separation of the lobe and disc
E	Concavity of the disc (Elliptical disc)

Device embolization typically occurs immediately after release and can most often be managed by percutaneous retrieval.[20] The site of embolization often relates to the closure device size, with larger devices more likely to remain in the left atrium or ventricle, whereas smaller occluders often migrate toward the descending aorta. A long sheath ≥2F larger than the device delivery sheath is required as well as the use of a snare and/or biotome to secure and withdraw the device into the sheath.[16] Depending on the location of the device, arterial access can be necessary. The most commonly used closure devices have retrieval techniques described: The WATCHMAN device is best captured by the distal frame struts, whereas the Amulet device can best be held at the central screw of the lobe as the delivery screw is recessed.[20] In general, retrieval is most simple from the aorta and more challenging from the left atrium (LA). Caution is advised if the device is lodged in the left ventricle and, in particular, in the mitral valve apparatus: surgery is often indicated in this instance.[20] Following device embolization and percutaneous retrieval, it may be reasonable to reattempt LAAC device implantation with updated TEE and/or CT sizing measurements and consideration of an alternative device size and/or position.

Periprocedural Stroke

Given that the purpose of the LAAC procedure is to prevent stroke, mitigation of procedural thromboembolic risk is vital. Procedural stroke rates of approximately 1% are noted across a range of studies and device types and have not changed over time.[1,10,21]

Ischemic periprocedural stroke is most often caused by embolism from thrombus formation in the relatively large delivery systems (12–14F) that are currently used during LAAC procedures. In addition, thrombus from the left atrium or its appendage can be dislodged during manipulation of the delivery system and device; therefore, it is strongly recommended to screen for thrombus by echocardiography before performing the transseptal puncture. To minimize the risk of thrombus formation, heparin administration with an initial dose of 100 IU/kg with a target procedural activated clotting time of greater than 250 seconds is advised. The option of administration of a part of this heparin dose before transseptal puncture can be considered.[12] Thrombus is occasionally noted on the delivery system by TEE and should prompt thorough aspiration. In addition, thrombolysis can be considered for de novo thrombus, which cannot be removed from the LA.[20] In case of periprocedural stroke, a cerebral angio-CT and cerebral clot retrieval/aspiration should be considered.

Given the documented rate of periprocedural stroke, it may be reasonable to use a cerebral embolic protection (CEP) device during LAAC. Despite similar stroke risk to TAVR (0.5%– 1.2%),[22,23] there remains relatively low uptake of CEP with LAAC procedures. Reluctance to use CEP is likely due to the lack of robust evidence in the setting of LAAC. However, small studies indicate the feasibility of this approach.[24]

Patients with thrombus present before LAAC are advised to complete 4 to 6 weeks of oral anticoagulant therapy and have a repeated imaging evaluation before LAAC. In rare instances, LAA thrombus may be refractory to anticoagulant therapy or patients may be unable to tolerate any length of oral anticoagulant therapy. Therefore, the potential to treat patients with LAAC, despite the presence of LAA thrombus, has been raised. One observational study found the rate of periprocedural complications, including stroke, was not different between patients with (n = 10) and without (n = 132) LAA thrombus present during LAAC.[25] Another series of 28 patients with LAA thrombus present during LAAC showed no major periprocedurally adverse embolic outcomes.[26] Caution should be taken with interpretation of these data because of the small number of cases; however, percutaneous LAAC in the presence of LAA thrombus is potentially an option for those high-risk patients for whom there is no alternative thromboembolic protection, and the use of a CEP device should always be considered in such cases as well as avoidance of delivery system manipulation deep in the LAA.

Air Embolus

Air embolus may cause stroke[1] and is commonly related to 2 sources. First, the delivery catheter is positioned in the low-pressure LA, where small decreases in intrathoracic pressure can cause atmospheric air to be drawn into the left heart. This risk is minimized by positioning the proximal end of the delivery catheter below the level of the left atrium and confirming by bleed-back that the delivery sheath is not sealed against the atrial wall, which may lead to vacuum formation during wire and introducer removal. Second, careful deairing of the device occluder is required before introduction. In either instance, the use of radiographic contrast in the delivery catheter during advancement of the LAA occluder can assist in the identification of air in the delivery system and also confirm the correctly maintained position of the delivery catheter relative to the LAA.[12]

Air embolism may present itself by acute hemodynamic instability or neurologic status alteration. In the supine position, the origin of the right coronary artery lies superiorly, and ischemic electrocardiogram changes may be noted in the inferior leads. In general, basic supportive care is required to support the patient with hyperbaric oxygen administration.[27] The LAA often lies superiorly as well, and air may persist here if introduced, being visible on fluoroscopy. Aspiration of air from the LAA via the delivery catheter system or pigtail catheter has been described.[20] Alternatively, prolonged supine bed rest of several hours may allow resorption of the collected air.[20]

POSTPROCEDURAL COMPLICATIONS

Late complications of LAAC have been defined as occurring more than 7 days after procedure[1,9] and relate to the integration of the device within the LAA.

Peridevice Leak

Peridevice leak is a common observation, noted in 10% to 33% of cases at postprocedural imaging follow-up.[10,28] Factors that impact the likelihood of incomplete LAAC include undersizing or oversizing of the closure device, device malposition or migration, a shallow (off-axis) closure device implantation, a highly elliptical LAA orifice, and incomplete endothelialization.[20] Gradation of peridevice leaks is arbitrary and based on early LAAC trial protocols; trivial (<1 mm), mild (1-3 mm), or significant (≥3-5 mm),[10,29] although no correlation between the size of the leak and adverse clinical outcomes, including stroke or systemic embolic events, has been demonstrated.[30] However, patients with incomplete closure are more likely to remain on anticoagulants,[28] negating the use of LAAC for many patients who undergo the procedure. In addition, there remains a high suspicion

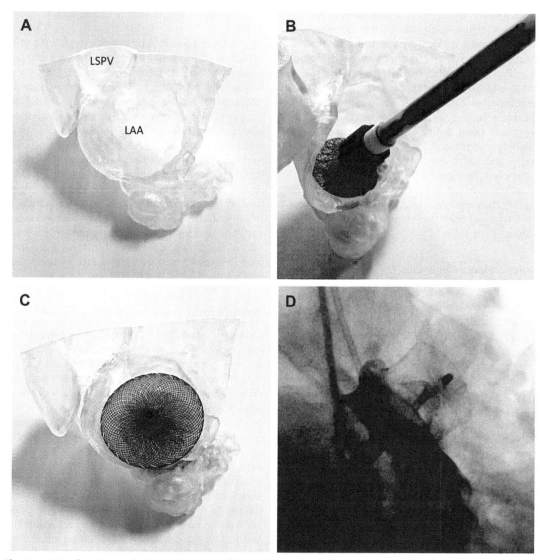

Fig. 1. LAAC planning and device sizing via 3D modeling. (*A*) Patient LAA 3D-printed model in silicone. (*B*) Deployment of LAAC device. (*C*) Assessment of device fit and position. (*D*) Implantation of predicted device size in vivo showing satisfactory LAA occlusion. LSPV, left superior pulmonary vein.

that an incompletely closed LAA can remain thrombogenic over the patient's lifetime.

The incidence of peridevice leak can be minimized with optimal device (size) selection and implantation technique. Additional preprocedural planning tools, such as patient-specific 3-dimensional (3D)-printed LAA models or computational modeling, are increasingly being used and may contribute to a better rate of complete LAAC (**Fig. 1**), although trials investigating the added value of these techniques are still on-going.[31]

An increasing number of LAAC procedures are currently being performed in local anesthetic with the use of ICE instead of TEE. A recent metaanalysis comparing procedural ICE to TEE showed no difference between the rates of procedural success, device embolization, and pericardial tamponade.[32] The ICE catheter can be used in the right heart and main pulmonary artery, or even better, crossed into the left atrium and PVs to generate procedural images; however, this does not fully compensate for the lack of multiplanar views available with TEE. Hence, ICE has a more limited ability to exclude the presence of important peridevice leak. Fluoroscopic assessment for safe device positioning, compression, and contrast assessment for peridevice leak remains needed in such setting.[12]

Small peridevice leak is likely to resolve following device endothelialization, and observational follow-up imaging is reasonable. Large peridevice leak will not disappear with time and may confer greater thrombotic risk because of the risk of larger organized thrombus escaping the low-flow LAA. It is possible to manage large peridevice leak via a secondary percutaneous closure procedure with generally safe and effective results.[30,33] A range of devices has been used to close the residual defect, including additional LAAC devices, vascular plugs, and atrial septal occluders.[33] Alternatively, continued oral anticoagulant therapy can be offered to patients with large peridevice leak, if they can tolerate oral anticoagulation, with reevaluation for closure after a few months.[20]

Device-Related Thrombus

Formation of device-related thrombus (DRT) is a potential complication of LAAC, especially early after implant before endothelization of the device. The incidence of DRT is generally reported to be 2% to 5% in previous cohorts.[10,34–37] Recent follow-up data of the AMPLATZER Amulet device showed that the DRT rate was 1.7% per year.[38] High CHADS2/CHA$_2$DS$_2$-VASc score, low ejection fraction, deep implantation of device, and incomplete LAA occlusion were reported to be risk factors for DRT.[2,39,40] Recent analyses found that large LAA width was also a significant predictor of DRT in cases of both WATCHMAN[39] and AMPLATZER Amulet devices.[40] Furthermore, the AMPLATZER Amulet device showed that most DRTs developed near the superior edge of the disc, close to the PV ridge, suggesting an uncovered PV ridge as a potential contributing factor for DRT.[38] Thus, to reduce the risk of DRT formation, the adequate closure device size should be chosen, especially in case of a large-size LAA, trying to avoid deep implantation and a large gap between the PV ridge and the device.

Previous studies evaluating WATCHMAN[34] and AMPLATZER[35] devices have reported no occurrence of stroke events in patients with DRT, or rates similar to those patients without DRT. On the other hand, a more recent report using prospective data from 4 Food and Drug Administration clinical trials reporting on the WATCHMAN device suggest an increased risk of thromboembolic events in patients with DRT.[37] Similarly, an analysis of the prospective Amulet Observational Study also showed that patients with a DRT were at a greater risk for ischemic stroke or transient ischemic attack as compared with non-DRT patients.[38] Therefore, DRT following LAAC needs

appropriate management to avoid future stroke events.

Current antithrombotic recommendations after LAAC vary between the types of devices and between centers. Ideal antithrombotic therapy in terms of preventing DRT remains unclear, although a recent propensity score matching for WATCHMAN revealed that initial OAC therapy is associated with a lower rate of DRT than antiplatelet therapy.[41] Similarly, there is no current consensus on the management strategy for DRT. However, anticoagulation using OAC or low-molecular-weight heparin could be used as first-line therapy in clinical practice. Although treatment duration varied greatly with reported minimal duration of 2 weeks and maximum duration of 6 months, complete thrombus resolution was achieved in 95% of cases with these strategies.[42]

Device Erosion/Late Pericardial Effusion

As experience with LAAC matures, a better long-term safety profile of the device in situ seems to be emerging, and late device complications are rare.[29] However, the most commonly used devices with long-term follow-up have reports of late erosion of the LAA or main pulmonary artery presenting with pericardial tamponade or death, occurring from several weeks to many months after implantation.[43,44] Late erosive complications have an alternative cause to the pericardial effusions that are noted periprocedurally. Unlike early pericardial effusion, caused by direct trauma to the atrium during deployment, erosion is likely caused by sustained local pressure exerted by the device on surrounding structures. Device erosion is presumably more likely with device oversizing and/or close apposition of the main pulmonary artery to the LAA, although no data exist on this topic.[45] The incidence of late device erosion and pericardial tamponade is low; an Italian registry of AMPLATZER cardiac plug cases has reported a mean follow-up period of 680 days for 134 patients post-LAAC. No perforation or erosion was observed in this group, and all patients had appropriate investigation to exclude late device-related complications or pericardial tamponade.[46] The presentation requires rapid assessment and management of any pericardial tamponade. In cases whereby bleeding persists, exploration and surgical hemostasis via collagen patch may be required. Cardiac CT has been used to locate the source of bleeding and has highlighted the close anatomic relationship of the LAA and the main pulmonary artery with this pathology.[45]

Table 1
Left atrial appendage closure complications: frequency, cause, prevention, and treatment options

	Frequency, %	Cause	Prevention	Treatment Options
Vascular complications	Up to 8.6	Local vascular trauma Large-caliber delivery system	US-guided access Closure device or figure-of -8 suture	Specific to complication
Transseptal puncture complications	1	Local trauma Inadequate septal visualization	TEE or ICE guidance Pigtail catheter at aortic root Puncture with RF energy	Repositioning of puncture site
Pericardial effusion	1–2	Transseptal puncture Local trauma to LA/LAA Device erosion	Minimize manipulations and excessive push Appropriate device sizing	Observation Deployment of device Percutaneous or surgical drainage
Device embolization	0.2–1	Device malposition or malalignment Inappropriate device size Unsuitable anatomy	Optimal device size Use device deployment criteria (if applicable) Stable "tug test"	Percutaneous or surgical device retrieval
Periprocedural stroke	0.1–1	Inadequate anticoagulation Large-caliber delivery system Preexisting LAA thrombus	ACT >250 s Minimize procedure duration Preprocedural identification of LAA thrombus Use of CEP	Delivery system aspiration Thrombolysis Consider cerebral clot retrieval
Air embolus	1	Air drawn into delivery system Incomplete device flush	Maintain delivery system below left heart when open Careful device flushing.	Supportive cares Hyperbaric O_2 Intravascular air aspiration (if feasible)
Device-related thrombus	1.7–5	Deep device implantation Incomplete sealing of LAA ostium	Optimal sealing of LAA ostium Consider early use of oral anticoagulants if tolerated	OAC or low-molecular-weight heparin

Abbreviation: RF, radiofrequency.

SUMMARY

LAAC has emerged as a promising therapy for thromboembolic prophylaxis in NVAF, particularly for patients at high bleeding risk during OAC. With increased experience and better preprocedural planning, the rates of periprocedural and postprocedural complications have been reduced. However, it is essential for LAAC operators to understand the potential procedural pitfalls, avoid complications though careful procedural planning and safe procedural execution, and know how to recognize and treat complications appropriately (**Table 1**).

ACKNOWLEDGEMENT

Dr Wilkins is supported by a grant from the Heart Foundation of New Zealand [Grant 1778].

DISCLOSURE

L. Søndergaard has received consultant fees and institutional research grants from Abbott and Boston Scientific. O. De Backer has been a consultant for Abbott and Boston Scientific. B. Wilkins and M. Fukutomi have no conflicts of interest to disclose.

REFERENCES

1. Holmes DR, Reddy VY, Turi ZG, et al. Percutaneous closure of the left atrial appendage versus warfarin therapy for prevention of stroke in patients with atrial fibrillation: a randomised non-inferiority trial. Lancet 2009;374:534–42.
2. Holmes DR Jr, Kar S, Price MJ, et al. Prospective randomized evaluation of the Watchman left atrial appendage closure device in patients with atrial fibrillation versus long-term warfarin therapy: the PREVAIL trial. J Am Coll Cardiol 2014;64:1–12.
3. Bungard TJ, Ghali WA, Teo KK, et al. Why do patients with atrial fibrillation not receive warfarin? Arch Intern Med 2000;160:41–6.
4. Landmesser U, Holmes DR Jr. Left atrial appendage closure: a percutaneous transcatheter approach for stroke prevention in atrial fibrillation. Eur Heart J 2012;33:698–704.
5. Bajaj NS, Parashar A, Agarwal S, et al. Percutaneous left atrial appendage occlusion for stroke prophylaxis in nonvalvular atrial fibrillation: a systematic review and analysis of observational studies. JACC Cardiovasc Interv 2014;7:296–304.
6. Sobolev M, Shiloh AL, Di Biase L, et al. Ultrasound-guided cannulation of the femoral vein in electrophysiological procedures: a systematic review and meta-analysis. Europace 2017;19:850–5.
7. Tanaka-Esposito CC, Chung MK, Abraham JM, et al. Real-time ultrasound guidance reduces total and major vascular complications in patients undergoing pulmonary vein antral isolation on therapeutic warfarin. J Interv Card Electrophysiol 2013;37:163–8.
8. Mohanty S, Trivedi C, Beheiry S, et al. Venous access-site closure with vascular closure device vs. manual compression in patients undergoing catheter ablation or left atrial appendage occlusion under uninterrupted anticoagulation: a multicentre experience on efficacy and complications. Europace 2019;21(7):1048–54.
9. Boersma LV, Schmidt B, Betts TR, et al. Implant success and safety of left atrial appendage closure with the WATCHMAN device: peri-procedural outcomes from the EWOLUTION registry. Eur Heart J 2016; 37:2465–74.
10. Tzikas A, Shakir S, Gafoor S, et al. Left atrial appendage occlusion for stroke prevention in atrial fibrillation: multicentre experience with the AMPLATZER cardiac plug. EuroIntervention 2016;11:1170–9.
11. Berti S, Santoro G, Brscic E, et al. Left atrial appendage closure using AMPLATZER devices: a large, multicenter, Italian registry. Int J Cardiol 2017;248:103–7.
12. Tzikas A, Gafoor S, Meerkin D, et al. Left atrial appendage occlusion with the AMPLATZER Amulet device: an expert consensus step-by-step approach. EuroIntervention 2016;11:1512–21.
13. Eng MH, Wang DD, Greenbaum AB, et al. Prospective, randomized comparison of 3-dimensional computed tomography guidance versus TEE data for left atrial appendage occlusion (PRO3DLAAO) 2018;92:401–7.
14. Reddy VY, Holmes D, Doshi SK, et al. Safety of percutaneous left atrial appendage closure: results from the Watchman Left Atrial Appendage System for Embolic Protection in Patients with AF (PROTECT AF) clinical trial and the continued access registry. Circulation 2011;123:417–24.
15. Price MJ. Prevention and management of complications of left atrial appendage closure devices. Interv Cardiol Clin 2014;3:301–11.
16. Saw J, Lempereur M. Percutaneous left atrial appendage closure: procedural techniques and outcomes. JACC Cardiovasc Interv 2014;7:1205–20.
17. Jazayeri MA, Vuddanda V, Parikh V, et al. Percutaneous left atrial appendage closure: current state of the art. Curr Opin Cardiol 2017;32:27–38.
18. Freixa X, Tzikas A, Basmadjian A, et al. The chicken-wing morphology: an anatomical challenge for left atrial appendage occlusion. J Interv Cardiol 2013; 26:509–14.
19. Apostolos T, Sameer G, David M, et al. Left atrial appendage occlusion with the AMPLATZER Amulet device: an expert consensus step-by-step approach. EuroIntervention 2016;11:1512–21.
20. Thakkar J, Vasdeki D, Tzikas A, et al. Incidence, prevention, and management of periprocedural complications of left atrial appendage occlusion. Interv Cardiol Clin 2018;7:243–52.
21. Reddy VY, Gibson DN, Kar S, et al. Post-approval U.S. experience with left atrial appendage closure for stroke prevention in atrial fibrillation. J Am Coll Cardiol 2017;69:253–61.
22. Popma JJ, Deeb GM, Yakubov SJ, et al. Transcatheter aortic-valve replacement with a self-expanding valve in low-risk patients. N Engl J Med 2019;380:1706–15.
23. Mack MJ, Leon MB, Thourani VH, et al. Transcatheter aortic-valve replacement with a balloon-expandable valve in low-risk patients. N Engl J Med 2019;380:1695–705.
24. Meincke F, Spangenberg T, Kreidel F, et al. Rationale of cerebral protection devices in left atrial

appendage occlusion. Catheter Cardiovasc Interv 2017;89:154–8.

25. Lee OH, Kim JS, Pak HN, et al. Feasibility of left atrial appendage occlusion for left atrial appendage thrombus in patients with persistent atrial fibrillation. Am J Cardiol 2018;121:1534–9.

26. Tarantini G, D'Amico G, Latib A, et al. Percutaneous left atrial appendage occlusion in patients with atrial fibrillation and left appendage thrombus: feasibility, safety and clinical efficacy. EuroIntervention 2018; 13:1595–602.

27. Casu G, Gulizia MM, Molon G, et al. ANMCO/AIAC/ SICI-GISE/SIC/SICCH consensus document: percutaneous occlusion of the left atrial appendage in non-valvular atrial fibrillation patients: indications, patient selection, staff skills, organisation, and training. Eur Heart J supplements 2017;19: D333–53.

28. Viles-Gonzalez JF, Kar S, Douglas P, et al. The clinical impact of incomplete left atrial appendage closure with the Watchman device in patients with atrial fibrillation: a PROTECT AF (Percutaneous Closure of the Left Atrial Appendage Versus Warfarin Therapy for Prevention of Stroke in Patients With Atrial Fibrillation) substudy. J Am Coll Cardiol 2012;59:923–9.

29. Reddy VY, Doshi SK, Kar S, et al. 5-year outcomes after left atrial appendage closure: from the PRE-VAIL and PROTECT AF trials. J Am Coll Cardiol 2017;70:2964–75.

30. Claire ER, Paul AF, Jacqueline S, et al. Residual leaks following percutaneous left atrial appendage occlusion: assessment and management implications. EuroIntervention 2017;13:1218–25.

31. Bieliauskas G, Otton J, Chow DHF, et al. Use of 3-dimensional models to optimize pre-procedural planning of percutaneous left atrial appendage closure. JACC Cardiovasc Interv 2017;10:1067–70.

32. Velagapudi P, Turagam MK, Kolte D, et al. Intracardiac vs transesophageal echocardiography for percutaneous left atrial appendage occlusion: a meta analysis. J Cardiovasc Electrophysiol 2019;30:461–7.

33. Hornung M, Gafoor S, Id D, et al. Catheter-based closure of residual leaks after percutaneous occlusion of the left atrial appendage. Catheter Cardiovasc Interv 2016;87:1324–30.

34. Boersma LV, Ince H, Kische S, et al. Efficacy and safety of left atrial appendage closure with WATCHMAN in patients with or without contraindication to oral anticoagulation: 1-year follow-up outcome data of the EWOLUTION trial. Heart Rhythm 2017;14:1302–8.

35. Saw J, Tzikas A, Shakir S, et al. Incidence and clinical impact of device-associated thrombus and peri-device leak following left atrial appendage closure with the amplatzer cardiac plug. JACC Cardiovasc Interv 2017;10:391–9.

36. Cochet H, Iriart X, Sridi S, et al. Left atrial appendage patency and device-related thrombus after percutaneous left atrial appendage occlusion: a computed tomography study. Eur Heart J Cardiovasc Imaging 2018;19:1351–61.

37. Dukkipati SR, Kar S, Holmes DR, et al. Device-related thrombus after left atrial appendage closure. Circulation 2018;138:874–85.

38. Aminian A, Schmidt B, Mazzone P, et al. Incidence, characterization, and clinical impact of device-related thrombus following left atrial appendage occlusion in the prospective global AMPLATZER amulet observational study. JACC Cardiovasc Interv 2019;12:1003–14.

39. Plicht B, Konorza TF, Kahlert P, et al. Risk factors for thrombus formation on the Amplatzer Cardiac Plug after left atrial appendage occlusion. JACC Cardiovasc Interv 2013;6:606–13.

40. Kar S, Hou D, Jones R, et al. Impact of Watchman and Amplatzer devices on left atrial appendage adjacent structures and healing response in a canine model. JACC Cardiovasc Interv 2014;7: 801–9.

41. Sondergaard L, Wong YH, Reddy VY, et al. Propensity-matched comparison of oral anticoagulation versus antiplatelet therapy after left atrial appendage closure with WATCHMAN. JACC Cardiovasc Interv 2019;12:1055–63.

42. Lempereur M, Aminian A, Freixa X, et al. Device-associated thrombus formation after left atrial appendage occlusion: a systematic review of events reported with the Watchman, the Amplatzer Cardiac Plug and the Amulet. Catheter Cardiovasc interv 2017;90:E111–21.

43. Wang E, Lin WW, Xu XF, et al. Delayed presentation of pulmonary artery perforation by an Amulet left atrial appendage closure device. BMJ Case Rep 2018;2018 [pii:bcr-2018-227098].

44. Scpahpour A, Ng MK, Storcy P, et al. Death from pulmonary artery erosion complicating implantation of percutaneous left atrial appendage occlusion device. Heart rhythm 2013;10:1810–1.

45. Halkin A, Cohen C, Rosso R, et al. Left atrial appendage and pulmonary artery anatomic relationship by cardiac-gated computed tomography: implications for late pulmonary artery perforation by left atrial appendage closure devices. Heart rhythm 2016;13:2064–9.

46. Santoro G, Meucci F, Stolcova M, et al. Percutaneous left atrial appendage occlusion in patients with non-valvular atrial fibrillation: implantation and up to four years follow-up of the AMPLATZER cardiac plug. EuroIntervention 2016;11:1188–94.

Postprocedural Management
Anticoagulation and Beyond

Moniek Maarse, MD[a],*, Martin J. Swaans, MD, PhD[a],
Lucas V.A. Boersma, MD, PhD[a,b]

KEYWORDS

- Left atrial appendage closure • Oral anticoagulation • Anti-platelet therapy
- Device related thrombus • Thromboembolic complications • Stroke

KEY POINTS

- The endothelialization phase of the left atrial appendage closure device is a vulnerable period of time when device-related thrombus/thromboembolic complications might occur, requiring adequate antithrombotic treatment.
- Initial protocol treatment after left atrial appendage closure with 45 days of warfarin combined with aspirin, 6 months of dual antiplatelet therapy, followed by lifelong aspirin was proven safe and efficient.
- Many left atrial appendage closure-treated patients are currently ineligible for warfarin; therefore, less intensive antithrombotic therapies were developed. To date only observational data are available.
- A tailored treatment, considering bleeding and thromboembolic risk based on patient/procedural characteristics in every patient, is probably the best approach.

INTRODUCTION

Left atrial appendage closure (LAAC) is an emerging alternative to oral anticoagulation (OAC) therapy for stroke prevention in patients with atrial fibrillation (AF) and increased risk for thromboembolic complications. Excluding the left atrial appendage (LAA), the main source of thrombi (>90%) in patients with nonvalvular AF,[1] is a mechanical approach to decrease stroke risk significantly, avoiding the risk of bleeding complications associated with long-term OAC therapy. Similar to other implanted cardiac devices (eg, coronary artery stents, patent foramen ovale closure devices) there is a time frame during the endothelialization period in which the foreign material of an LAAC device is exposed to circulating blood, which can activate the coagulation cascade. Although this step is essential for the healing process of the LAAC device, in excessive proportions it might result in the development of device-related thrombus (DRT) and possibly thromboembolic complications. This vulnerable time frame requires a bridging period with optimal antithrombotic drug therapy. However, such therapies have the risk of causing bleeding complications, especially in the target population for LAAC with contraindications to anticoagulation. A carefully balanced approach is required, preventing thromboembolic complications, as well as avoiding an increase of bleeding complications.

This review addresses the critical topic of post-LAAC medical treatment options described in the literature. In addition, relationships

[a] Department of Cardiology, St. Antonius Hospital, Koekoekslaan 1, 3435CM Nieuwegein, The Netherlands;
[b] Department of Cardiology, Amsterdam UMC, Meibergdreef 9, 1105 AZ Amsterdam, The Netherlands
* Corresponding author.
E-mail address: m.maarse@antoniusziekenhuis.nl

Card Electrophysiol Clin 12 (2020) 77–88
https://doi.org/10.1016/j.ccep.2019.10.002
1877-9182/20/© 2019 Elsevier Inc. All rights reserved.

between various post-LAAC treatments and thromboembolic/bleeding complications are summarized. Last, the future perspectives of post-LAAC medical treatment is evaluated. This review focuses on the most commonly used devices in percutaneous LAAC, being the WATCHMAN (WM), AMPLATZER Cardiac Plug (ACP), and AMPLATZER Amulet, because there is only limited experience with several other newer devices.

ENDOTHELIALIZATION

The endothelialization period of LAAC devices has been investigated in small experimental canine studies. Kar and colleagues[2] observed complete neo-endocardial coverage of WM devices implanted in 3 canines after 28 days after implantation during administration of warfarin combined with aspirin. The other 3 canines implanted with ACP devices still had some focal uncovered areas of the device. Another study implanted 10 ACP devices in canines and sacrificed the canines 90 days after implantation. Histologically, all ACP devices showed stable mature neointima on the complete surface while the canines received aspirin throughout the whole study period.[3] A third study evaluated the healing process after WM implantation histopathologically in 9 canines at different time points: 3 days, 45 days and 90 days after implantation. At 3 days, a small layer of organizing thrombus covered the prosthetic device. After 45 days, granulation tissue had developed with a thin layer of endothelial-like cells covering the complete device, whereas the prior thrombus deposition was replaced by endocardium surrounded by mild inflammation. After 90 days, the former LAA ostium was completely covered by endocardial lining, organizing thrombus had completely transformed to connective tissue, and inflammation tissue had disappeared. In the same study, 4 human hearts (>139 days after implantation) of patients who died of causes unrelated to the device or procedure were studied. Resemblance of device endothelialization of the investigated canines was shown, although variability in organized neo-endocardial coverage was observed. Compared with the healing process in animals, human healing seems to take more time and may vary between patients.[4] Previously described durations of intensified post-LAAC antithrombotic regimens vary from 1 to 6 months and are based on the assumption that endothelialization is completed after this period of time, although it is uncertain if and after how much time complete endothelialization can be assumed.

The vulnerable endothelialization period after LAAC shows many similarities with other, longer existing, cardiac implants (eg, coronary artery stents, patent foramen ovale occluders), and therefore postprocedural LAAC antithrombotic regimen was partially adopted from the experience gained with these cardiac devices. Investigation of the thrombosis mechanisms in these devices showed the importance of platelet-induced thrombus growth, emphasizing the importance of antiplatelet therapy.[5] Early clinical trials investigating coronary artery stenting showed high rates of stent thrombosis ($\leq$20%), resulting in the need for an adequate antithrombotic regimen, eventually leading to the wide acceptance of dual antiplatelet therapy (DAPT).[6] However, the ongoing debate regarding optimal DAPT duration reflects the therapeutic dilemma of optimal antithrombotic treatment without increasing major bleeding complications similar to the dilemma in after LAAC treatment.

INITIAL PROTOCOL TREATMENT

The WM device is the only percutaneous LAAC device investigated in randomized, controlled trials that is, the PROTECT-AF[7] and PREVAIL[8] studies. These studies revealed noninferiority of LAAC to warfarin therapy in the prevention of stroke in patients with nonvalvular AF. All patients enrolled in both studies were eligible for warfarin and a strict postprocedural medical treatment was pursued to overcome the initial vulnerable phase during endothelialization of the device. Directly after LAAC, a 45-day continuation of warfarin therapy combined with aspirin (81 mg) was advised. Afterward, when follow-up imaging by transesophageal echocardiography confirmed complete closure and no DRT, DAPT with aspirin (81–325 mg) and clopidogrel (75 mg) was prescribed for the following 6 months. If no thromboembolic events occurred, indefinite aspirin (325 mg) was the final and chronic treatment. After approval by the US Food and Drug Administration of the WM device in 2015, the use of this alternative to long-term OAC therapy has gained ground in clinical practice, although the indication for LAAC and therefore patient characteristics of with LAAC treated patients vary substantially. In the United States, patients with a good reason to seek an alternative to OAC may be indicated for LAAC, and the original antithrombotic drug therapy is still mandated by the US Food and Drug Administration. This actually makes it difficult to implant the device in patients with a strict contraindication to (novel) OAC ([N]OAC) treatment, because it subjects such patients to a higher bleeding risk during

45 days of combined (N)OAC plus aspirin, and DAPT up to 6 months. It is unclear how exactly such patients are currently managed in everyday clinical practice. In European guidelines, LAAC is only recommended for patients who are intolerant or contraindicated to long-term OAC therapy (Class IIb, Level of Evidence B), although this population has never been represented in any randomized trial investigating LAAC.[9] As a result, the vast majority of patients currently being treated with LAAC are patients who previously experienced a major bleeding complication, for example, intracranial hemorrhage or major gastrointestinal bleedings. Postprocedural management prescribed in the PROTECT-AF and PREVAIL trials, therefore, needed adjustment because many of these patients are deemed unsuitable for this intensified antithrombotic regimen. Observational evidence available shows a wide variety of postprocedural antithrombotic treatment options; however, optimal therapy remains challenging and is highly determined by individual patient comorbidity, while randomized trial evidence regarding this issue is lacking. Less aggressive antithrombotic postprocedural LAAC therapies would be appealing, potentially causing less bleeding complications, which to this date is the most common and challenging complication after LAAC.

THROMBOEMBOLIC EVENTS AND BLEEDING COMPLICATIONS

An overview of the most relevant and influencing studies, which evaluated the effectiveness and safety of the post-LAAC medical treatment, is discussed. **Table 1** and **Fig. 1** summarize the outcomes of these studies regarding thromboembolic and bleeding complications after LAAC. **Fig. 2** illustrates the most relevant antithrombotic strategies encountered in currently available literature.

ORAL ANTICOAGULATION AND ANTIPLATELET THERAPY (TREATMENT A)

Most solid evidence for effective post-LAAC antithrombotic therapy results from the earlier performed PROTECT-AF/PREVAIL trials and their continued access registries. Recently, the 5-year results of the combined PROTECT-AF and PREVAIL population (2:1 randomization; n = 732 in WM arm; 2850 patient-years of follow-up) were published and demonstrated a comparable combined rate of stroke and systemic embolism (SE) in the WM device group as compared with the warfarin group (hazard ratio [HR], 0.96; $P = .87$). Although the risk of ischemic stroke and SE were

numerically higher with LAAC, there was a significant decrease in hemorrhagic stroke (HR, 0.20; $P = .0022$) and major bleeding if procedure-related events were excluded (HR, 0.48; $P = .0003$).[10] Furthermore, Dukkipati and colleagues[11] studied the incidence and clinical outcomes of DRT in all patients included in the randomized PROTECT-AF/PREVAIL device arms plus the continued access registries, CAP-I and CAP-II together (n = 1739 patients; 7159 patient-years of follow-up). Seventy-four DRTs were observed in 65 patients (3.7%). DRT was associated with approximately a 3-fold increase of embolic events; however, the majority of patients with DRT (74%) did not experience stroke or SE and a temporal relationship was suspected in only one-half of the patients (using a 1-month window). Annual DRT rates were calculated for different time intervals after LAAC and seemed to decrease with increasing follow-up duration, confirming that most DRTs occur shortly after implantation. Nevertheless, DRT was not restricted to the initial phase of device endothelialization and was also observed more than 6 months after implantation. Delayed endothelialization and the cessation of antithrombotic treatment could potentially have provoked thrombus formation in these cases. A pooled patient analysis of PROTECT-AF and PREVAIL showed a comparable major bleeding rate between the device arm and warfarin arm, but in the device arm most events occurred directly after implantation and were procedure related.[12] LAAC decreased the rate of major bleedings substantially over time, especially after discontinuation of DAPT/OAC treatment. All these results confirm that the initial protocol is safe and efficient as post-LAAC treatment in patients eligible for warfarin use.

DUAL ANTIPLATELET THERAPY (TREATMENT B)

As a consequence of the shift of patients treated with LAAC toward patients not eligible for warfarin, DAPT directly after LAAC is now the most commonly used post-LAAC treatment option outside of the United States. The ASAP trial performed an analysis in 150 nonrandomized patients treated with WM LAAC who were considered ineligible for warfarin treatment. These patients were treated with DAPT for 6 months (ticlopidine or clopidogrel combined with aspirin) and continued with life-long aspirin. The observed low annualized stroke rate of 1.7% (>70% lower than expected without any treatment) and DRT rate of 4% were comparable with the device arms of the PROTECT-AF/PREVAIL, suggesting DAPT without

Table 1
Summary of most important previous published studies, their postprocedural antithrombotic and important outcomes

	PROTECT-AF[7,10,12]	PREVAIL[8,10,12]	ASAP[27]	ACP Registry[28]	Korsholm et al,[20] 2017	EWOLUTION[14]	RELEXAO[21]	Enomoto et al,[29] 2017	WASP[30]	Global Amulet Registry[31]
	2005–2008	2010–2012	2009–2011	2008–2013	2010–2015	2013–2015	2012–2017	2015–2016	2014–2015	2015–2016
Study design	RCT	RCT	Prospective registry	Prospective registry	Prospective registry	Prospective registry	Prospective registry	Prospective registry	Prospective registry	Prospective registry
No. of patients (successful implants)	463 (408) device arm	269 (252)	150 (142)	1047 (1019)	110 (107)	1025 (1005)	487 (469)	214 (214)	201 (198)	1088 (1078)
Follow-up duration	1782 patient-years	1043 patient-years	14.4 ± 8.6 mo 177 patient-years	13 [6–25] mo 1349 patient-years	2.3 [1.6–3.2] y 266 patient-years	732 [677–757] d	13 ± 13 mo	NA	684 ± 161 d	11.1 ± 2.6 mo
Device type	WM	WM	WM	ACP	ACP, Amulet	WM	WM, ACP, Amulet	WM	WM	Amulet
Post-LAAC antithrombotic therapy	45 d: Warfarin + ASA 6 mo: Clopidogrel + ASA Indefinite: ASA	45 d: Warfarin + ASA 6 mo: Clopidogrel + ASA Indefinite: ASA	6 mo: Clopidogrel/ticlopidine + ASA Indefinite: ASA	At discharge: (N)OAC + APT 10% (N)OAC 17% LMWH + APT 5% DAPT 16% SAPT 35% LMWH 7% None 8% Unknown 1%	At discharge: SAPT 88% DAPT 12%	At discharge N)OAC 27% DAPT 60% SAPT 7% None 6%	At discharge: (N)OAC + APT 4% (N)OAC 29% DAPT 23% SAPT 36% None 8%	At discharge: NOAC	At discharge: VKA 12% NOAC 47% DAPT 27% SAPT 11% None 4%	At discharge: (N)OAC + APT 7% (N)OAC 5% DAPT 58% SAPT 23% None 2% Other 5%
CHA_2DS	2.2 ± 1.2	2.6 ± 1.0	2.8 ± 1.2	2.8 ± 1.3	NA	2.8 ± 1.3	NA	2.1 ± 1.2	2.5 ± 1.4	NA
CHA_2DS_2-VASc	3.4 ± 1.5	4.0 ± 1.2	4.4 ± 1.7	4.4 ± 1.6	4.4 ± 1.6	4.5 ± 1.6	4.5 ± 1.4	3.8 ± 1.4	3.9 ± 1.7	4.2 ± 1.6

HAS-BLED	1.9 ± 0.9[b] (modified)	1.9 ± 0.9[b] (modified)	NA	3.1 ± 1.2	4.1 ± 1.1	2.3 ± 1.2	3.7 ± 1.0	2.4 ± 1.0	2.1 ± 1.2	3.3 ± 1.1
Observed annual rate stroke	1.4%	1.7%	.7%	1.3%	2.3%	1.3%	4.0%	NA	1.6%	2.9%
Expected annual rate stroke[a]	5.3%	6.4%	7.1%	7.1%	7.1%	7.2%	7.2%	6.0%	6.2%	6.7%
Observed annual rate stroke/ TIA/SE	NA	NA	NA	2.3%	NA	2.0%	NA	NA	1.9%	3.8%
Expected annual rate stroke/ TIA/SE[a]	7.5%	8.9%	9.9%	9.9%	9.9%	10.2%	10.2%	8.6%	8.7%	9.4%
Observed annual major bleeding rate	3.1%	3.1%	NA	2.1%	3.8%	2.7%	3.8%	NA	2.2%	10.3%
Expected annual major bleeding rate[a,c]	4.4%	4.4%	NA	6.4%	8.1%	5.0%	7.4%	5.2%	4%, 7%	6.7%

Abbreviations: APT, antiplatelet therapy; ASA, aspirin; LMWH, low-molecular-weight heparin; NA, not available; (N)OAC, (novel) oral anticoagulant; RCT, randomized controlled trial; SAPT, single antiplatelet therapy; SE, systemic embolism; TIA, transient ischemic attack; VKA, vitamin K antagonist.

[a] Expected annual scores were based on average HAS-BLED and CHA_2DS_2-VASc risk scores of the populations, extrapolated from published risk scores by Friberg and colleagues[31] (CHA_2DS_2-VASc adapted for aspirin) and Lip and colleagues[33] (HAS-BLED under OAC).

[b] Modified HAS-BLED scores were retrospectively calculated for the PROTECT-AF/PREVAIL based on the separate variables that were systematically collected (liver dysfunction and labile international normalized ratio variables were missing).

[c] Major bleeding was defined as BARC of ≥ 3.

Annual ischemic stroke rate

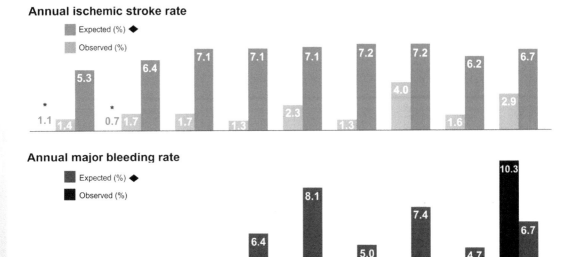

Annual major bleeding rate

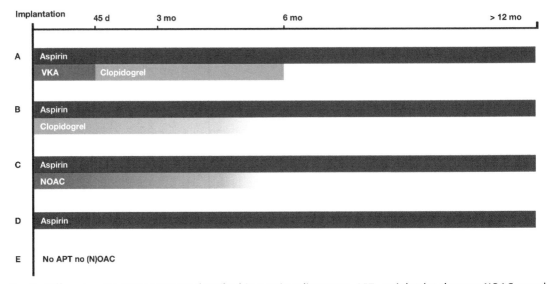

Fig. 1. Observed and expected annual rates of ischemic stroke and major bleeding. ◆ Expected annual scores were based on average HAS-BLED and CHA_2DS_2-VASc risk scores of the populations, extrapolated from published risk scores by Friberg and colleagues[32] (CHA_2DS_2-VASc adapted for aspirin) and Lip and colleagues[33] (HAS-BLED under OAC). * Warfarin arm. In PROTECT-AF/PREVAIL not only comparison to expected rates based on risk scores but also comparison to the warfarin arms is presented.

warfarin being a suitable option directly after LAAC.

Everyday clinical practice data presented by the largest prospective multicenter WM trial EWOLUTION showed DAPT as the most regularly allocated post-LAAC treatment in 60% of all patients. Within this trial, only 16% and 11% of patients were treated by vitamin K antagonists and direct NOACs, respectively.[13] At the end of the study, 85% of the patients were solely using single antiplatelet therapy (SAPT) or no antithrombotic treatment at all. Two-year follow-up data of the

Fig. 2. Different post-LAAC treatment described in previous literature. APT, antiplatelet therapy; NOAC, novel oral anticoagulant; VKA, vitamin K agonist.

EWOLUTION trial were recently presented and showed low annualized ischemic stroke rates of 1.3% and DRT in 2.8%, despite the investigated population being a high-risk patient group (mean age, 73.4 ± 8.9; CHA_2DS_2-VASc, 4.5 ± 1.6; HAS-BLED, 2.3 ± 1.2).[14] No association was found between DRT/ischemic events and the type of allocated antithrombotic treatment, although the numbers of patients in the various post-LAAC medical treatment groups were low and subject to selection bias. An association between DRT and annual rates of ischemic events was not observed. The incidence of bleeding events decreased over time in accordance with the results of the device arms of PROTECT-AF/PREVAIL.[12] Furthermore, a propensity-matched comparison of late (>105 days) versus early discontinuation of DAPT showed a trend favoring early discontinuation (bleeding rate 3.1% vs 1.1%; P = .122) without increasing thromboembolic events. Based on the data from the EWOLUTION trial, DAPT was admitted to the recommended anticoagulation scheme after LAAC in the instructions for use of the WM device outside of the United States. The prospective observational WASP registry, which was performed in the Asia-Pacific region, included 201 patients of whom almost 30% was treated with DAPT. The results of the WASP registry showed comparable results with the EWOLUTION trial with a 1.6% annual ischemic stroke rate, a 2.2% annual major bleeding rate, and a 2.5% DRT rate.

Concerning the AMPLATZER device, the other most common used catheter-based devices, DAPT treatment was already recommended at the time of introduction of this device on the market. These recommendations were based on the well-established AMPLATZER occluder technology used for other purposes (eg, patent foramen ovale or atrial septal defect). Although no randomized data are available, large observational studies have been performed. In the ACP registry (n = 1047), patients were treated with DAPT (16%) or SAPT (35%) and less frequently with vitamin K antagonists, NOACs and low-molecular-weight heparin. The 1-year results showed similarities with the earlier published WM data. The annual rates of ischemic stroke and major bleeding in the ACP registry were 1.3% and 2.1%, respectively, and DRT occurred in 2.7% of all patients. Most ischemic and bleeding events occurred early after the procedure, and these results suggest that the benefit of LAAC becomes more apparent with more prolonged follow-up time. Of note, in this study no correlation between DRT and ischemic events was described.

The global Amulet registry (n = 1088) published the results of the next generation of the ACP device, the AMPLATZER Amulet, in 2018. This registry demonstrated a slightly higher annual ischemic stroke rate of 2.9%, whereas the incidence of DRT (1.6% of all patients) remained low, despite the fact that most patients were using less aggressive antithrombotic (SAPT, no antithrombotics) regimen after LAAC. The annual major bleeding rate was 10.3%, which was substantially higher than in the EWOLUTION trial or ACP trial. This could partially be explained by a higher risk for major bleedings as depicted by the relatively high HAS-BLED score (mean, 3.3), the higher frequency of previous major bleeding complications before LAAC, and a shorter follow-up duration with most events occurring in the early phase after device implantation.

Recently, a propensity-matched comparison between patients post-LAAC treated with OAC (n = 1018; 95% warfarin and 5% NOAC) or APT (n = 509; 91% DAPT and 9% SAPT) was published.[15] No differences in major bleeding or thromboembolism during follow-up were observed; however, more patients in the APT treatment arm suffered from DRT (OAC 1.4% and APT 3.1%; P = .018). These results remained favorable after treatment with OAC if patients treated with SAPT and patients without follow-up imaging were excluded from the analysis. However, in the OAC group 3 patients with DRT experienced a thromboembolic complication and in the APT group no patients with DRT had thromboembolic complications. The similar clinically relevant event rates of this study support the wide acceptance of antiplatelet therapy as post-LAAC treatment. Of note, it is important to realize that the patient groups in this study remain substantially different irrespective of the propensity matching, owing to the fact that ineligibility for OAC treatment was the number one reason for administering APT.

Clopidogrel resistance is an interesting topic not often discussed in the previous LAAC literature, although possibly of influence in developing DRT. Ketterer and colleagues[16] reported a case series of 46 patients treated with LAAC of whom 4 patients developed DRT. Of these patients, 3 (75%) had clopidogrel resistance diagnosed by platelet function testing. Therefore, many patients may not even benefit from the addition of clopidogrel, and the benefit and need of DAPT to lower thrombosis may be overestimated. Data from Chun and colleagues[17] suggest that SAPT may be noninferior to DAPT for the risk of stroke and DRT. Whether modern single APT such as prasugrel or ticagrelor could facilitate optimal postprocedural antithrombotic management is currently unknown.

NOVEL ORAL ANTICOAGULANTS (TREATMENT C)

In the past decade, the NOACs have been developed and their usage in clinical practice has increased exponentially. Several meta-analyses evaluating the effectiveness of different NOACs compared with warfarin concerning stroke and SE prevention in patients with nonvalvular AF have been previously published. The results of these reports demonstrated reduced rates of stroke and SE comparable with warfarin. Moreover, lower intracranial hemorrhage and major bleeding events were described, making NOACs an appealing post-LAAC treatment option.[18] NOACs are not well-represented in currently available literature about post-LAAC treatment because the majority of studies were conducted before the widespread introduction of the NOACs. Enomoto and colleagues[29] conducted a study that did include NOACs as a post-LAAC treatment. The authors compared 214 patients treated with NOACs (46% apixaban, 46% rivaroxaban, 7% dabigatran, and 1% edoxaban) after LAAC with 212 patients receiving warfarin, showing comparable rates of DRT (0.9% vs 0.5%), and of a composite endpoint, including thromboembolism (1.4% vs 0.9%) and postprocedural bleeding events (0.5% vs 0.9%). The EWOLUTION trial also included a small group of patients treated with a NOAC after LAAC (n = 109), and no concerns were raised for the use of this post-LAAC regimen because no strokes were seen in the patient group treated with NOAC after 3 months of follow-up and the occurrence of DRT was not associated with post-LAAC antithrombotic regimens.[19] Although the body of evidence is scarce, the results from the study by Enomoto and colleagues[29] and the EWOLUTION trial may suggest that NOACs are feasible as post LAAC treatment. More studies investigating the efficacy and safety in this particular patient population are warranted. An appealing future post-LAAC treatment could be the (longer term) use of (low-dose) NOACs instead of (D)APT, potentially diminishing post-LAAC bleeding complications as well as the risk of thromboembolic events.

SINGLE ANTIPLATELET THERAPY OR NO ANTITHROMBOTIC TREATMENT (TREATMENTS D AND E)

In a select population category SAPT or no antithrombotic therapy is prescribed directly after LAAC. In these patients (N)OAC/DAPT treatment is often withheld owing to concerns of serious bleeding complications (eg, patients with Rendu Osler

Weber disease or with cerebral amyloid angiopathy). Despite a greater potential for thromboembolic complications, observational studies show variable outcomes. In the EWOLUTION trial, 7% and 6% of all patients were discharged on SAPT and no antithrombotic treatment, respectively. Despite the highest $CHAD_2S_2$-VASc scores in these patients (mean of 4.7 and 4.8) only 1 ischemic stroke was seen after 3 months of follow-up, and was comparable with other antithrombotic regimens (P = .5108).[19] Korsholm and colleagues[20] reported on 110 patients treated with aspirin alone after LAAC treatment. The annual ischemic stroke rate was 2.3% and DRT was observed in 1.9% of patients, whereas the annual risk of major bleeding was reduced by 57% in this high-risk bleeding population (mean HAS-BLED of 4.1 ± 1.1). These results suggest the potential feasibility of aspirin monotherapy after LAAC. However, the published results of the RELEXAO study did raise concerns regarding less aggressive antithrombotic regimens after LAAC.[21] After LAAC within this study, 36%, 8%, and 4% of patients received SAPT, no antithrombotic treatment, or combined OAC/APT, respectively, in accordance with the initial protocol treatment. In the whole cohort, DRT was observed in 5.5% of patients and the annual ischemic stroke rate was 4.0%, which were both higher than all previous reported studies in the literature. DAPT and OAC treatment after LAAC were associated with lower rates of DRT (DAPT: HR, 0.10 [P = .03] and OAC: HR, 0.26 [P = .02]), whereas DRT was an independent predictor for stroke/transient ischemic attack (HR, 4.4; P = .04). Thus, considering available data regarding SAPT or no antithrombotic treatment at all after LAAC treatment, additional evidence is required to draw any firm conclusions. Because an increasing number of patients treated with LAAC are at high risk for bleeding complications, this area is important for further research.

DEVICE-RELATED THROMBUS

In **Fig. 3**, DRT rates in prior literature about LAAC are summarized. Although DRT seems the most reasonable outcome to measure efficacy of post-LAAC treatment, we did encounter some difficulties. First, a lack of consensus on the definition of DRT may cause over-reporting or under-reporting of DRT. A fine laminar layer of thrombotic material on the device may be part of the healing process and not clinically relevant. Most studies omit to report their definition of DRT. An association between DRT and thromboembolic events has been rarely confirmed, indicating that

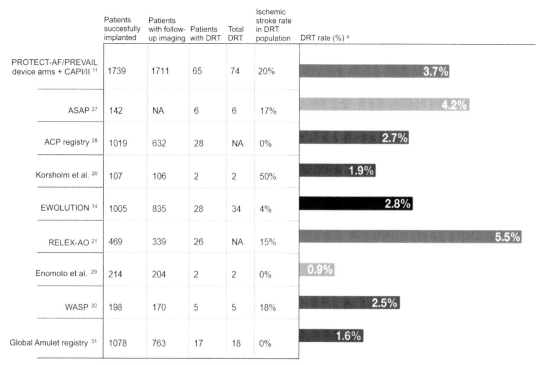

	Patients succesfully implanted	Patients with follow-up imaging	Patients with DRT	Total DRT	Ischemic stroke rate in DRT population	DRT rate (%) [a]
PROTECT-AF/PREVAIL device arms + CAPI/II [11]	1739	1711	65	74	20%	3.7%
ASAP [27]	142	NA	6	6	17%	4.2%
ACP registry [28]	1019	632	28	NA	0%	2.7%
Korsholm et al. [20]	107	106	2	2	50%	1.9%
EWOLUTION [14]	1005	835	28	34	4%	2.8%
RELEX-AO [21]	469	339	26	NA	15%	5.5%
Enomoto et al. [29]	214	204	2	2	0%	0.9%
WASP [30]	198	170	5	5	18%	2.5%
Global Amulet registry [31]	1078	763	17	18	0%	1.6%

Fig. 3. DRT in the most important previous published studies. [a] The rate of DRT is expressed as the number of patients with DRT divided by the total number of patients implanted with LAAC devices. NA, not available.

possible other sources for emboli may be responsible in these cases. DRT rates are often represented in different ways, making a comparison between studies difficult. Many studies do not report what kind of drug therapy was administered at the time of DRT diagnosis, and often there is insufficient imaging at the time of the event, which makes it challenging to assess the acute association between DRT and post-LAAC treatment. Furthermore, event rates strongly correlated with the frequency of imaging performed, hinting toward a substantial bias by indication. Important to recognize is that DRT development is probably multifactorial and patient and procedural characteristics may influence thromboembolic/bleeding outcomes. The risk for DRT has been described to be higher in patients with a lower left ventricular ejection fraction, large LAA, older age, prior stroke/transient ischemic attack, permanent AF, and vascular disease.[22] DRT has often been observed in patients with deeper implanted devices, which can result in the uncovering of the more proximal area on the LAA.[23] In addition, thrombi seemed to occur more often located at the central screw, an observation that has resulted in the development of a less protruding central screw in the newer generation WM Flex and Amplatzer Amulet.[24] Interestingly Lempereur and colleagues[23] provided a

meta-analysis on DRT after LAAC with the WM device, ACP device, and the Amplatzer Amulet. A total of 30 studies (2118 patients) were included and the overall incidence of DRT was 3.9%. Median time to DRT diagnosis was 1.5 months. Only 6 patients had thromboembolic complications associated with DRT and presented with transient ischemic attack (n = 4) or ischemic stroke (n = 2). Complete thrombus resolution was achieved in nearly all cases (95%) with intensified antithrombotic treatment (eg, low-molecular-weight heparin or reinitiating of OAC). Of note, intensifying antithrombotic therapy may lead to an increase of bleeding complications, although this outcome was never clearly described. Finally, although most DRT occur during the endothelialization phase, case reports about patients with very late (>10 years after implantation) DRT development have been described and possibly other mechanisms causing DRT are involved in these patients.[25]

FUTURE PERSPECTIVES

A consensus document about the optimal post-LAAC treatment strategy, duration of treatment, and the preferred imaging modality and timing after LAAC is currently not available. However, randomized studies further evaluating this intriguing issue are being conducted and may answer some of remaining concerns about the optimal post-LAAC treatment. The results of the randomized ADRIFT trial (NCT03273322) are the first to be expected; 105 patients will be randomized (1:1:1) to either rivaroxaban (10 or 15 mg) or DAPT treatment after LAAC. The aim is to investigate whether rivaroxaban is able to suppress coagulation after LAAC adequately. The CLOSURE-AF trial (NCT03463317) will randomize 1512 nonvalvular AF patients and will be due in 2023. The study investigates if DAPT treatment after LAAC is noninferior to the best medical care (including [N]OAC when eligible). The Amulet-IDE study (NCT02879448) will be the first to compare the 2 most commonly used devices: the WM device combined with an initial post-LAAC antithrombotic regimen, or the Amplatzer Amulet with DAPT as post-LAAC treatment. The randomized ASAP-TOO trial (NCT02928497) with patients with AF deemed ineligible for OAC will be comparing LAAC with post-LAAC APT with a control group receiving aspirin or no treatment at all.

Currently available evidence indicates that a shorter duration of intensified antithrombotic treatment is associated with lower bleeding rates, encouraging further diminishing and shortening of intensified antithrombotic regimens without increasing thromboembolic complications. Duration of aspirin use, initially prescribed lifelong after LAAC, is also questionable in patients with no vascular diseases or other indications requiring APT treatment. The effect of aspirin on bleeding events is not negligible and the effect on decreasing thromboembolic risk in patients with AF has never been demonstrated in a profound way, suggesting that aspirin treatment after complete endothelialization being possibly detrimental.[26]

Patients with thromboembolic complications, for example, ischemic stroke, treated by adequate OAC before LAAC is another interesting subgroup for future analysis, now often receiving post-LAAC treatments comparable with patients with high bleeding risks with gradually more conservative antithrombotic regimens. Possibly a future hybrid strategy of LAAC combined with continued (N)OAC could decrease stroke rates even further and should be evaluated in the future.

Finally, epicardial LAAC or novel endocardial closure devices constructed of nonthrombogenic material could diminish or abolish the need for antithrombotic therapy. The new WM FLX design with reduction of exposed thrombogenic metal is currently being introduced and may also decrease the need for postprocedural anticoagulation.

SUMMARY

Post-LAAC medical treatment with OAC and APT continued with DAPT after 45 days until 6 months after implantation has been proven safe and efficient in nonvalvular AF patients eligible for vitamin K antagonist treatment and treated with LAAC. However, in everyday clinical practice many patients are ineligible for warfarin use, even for a short period of time, and therefore this post-LAAC treatment is unsuitable. Other medical post-LAAC regimens in patients not eligible for warfarin were described in observational studies, although these treatments were and may never become compared in randomized trials. Real-world data show that DAPT is the most common used alternative directly after LAAC, showing similar outcomes regarding bleeding rates and ischemic complication rates compared with the initial protocol treatment. Observational data of diminishing bleeding rates after cessation of antithrombotic treatment encourages establishing even less aggressive treatments, for example, low-dose NOACs, SAPT, or no antithrombotic drug treatment at all. The possibility of a higher DRT rate and thromboembolic risk should not be underestimated, and requires further study.

Finding a one-size-fits-all optimal post-LAAC antithrombotic treatment is probably impossible because of the wide variety of comorbidities in LAAC-treated patients. A tailored treatment, considering bleeding and thromboembolic risk based on patient and procedural characteristics in every individual patient, is probably the best approach. The upcoming randomized studies will hopefully add valuable information, helping physicians in making more evidence-based decisions.

DISCLOSURE

M. Maarse, has no conflicts of interest to declare. L.V.A. Boersma is a consultant for Boston Scientific and proctor for Abbott. M.J. Swaans reports proctoring fees for training/educational services to the Department of Cardiology from Boston Scientific, and personal fees from Abbott, Philips Healthcare and Bioventrix Inc.

REFERENCES

1. Blackshear JL, Odell JA. Appendage obliteration to reduce stroke in cardiac surgical patients with atrial fibrillation. Ann Thorac Surg 1996;61:755–9.
2. Kar S, Hou D, Jones R, et al. Impact of WATCHMAN and Amplatzer devices on left atrial appendage adjacent structures and healing response in a canine model. JACC Cardiovasc Interv 2014;7(7): 801–9.

3. Bass JL. Transcatheter occlusion of the left atrial appendage-experimental testing of a new Amplatzer device. Catheter Cardiovasc Interv 2010;76(2):181–5.

4. Schwartz RS, Holmes DR, Van Tassel RA, et al. Left atrial appendage obliteration: mechanisms of healing and intracardiac integration. JACC Cardiovasc Interv 2010;3(8):870–7.

5. Polzin A, Dannenberg L, Sophia Popp V, et al. Antiplatelet effects of clopidogrel and aspirin after interventional patent foramen ovale/atrium septum defect closure. Platelets 2016;27(4):317–21.

6. Leon MB, Baim DS, Popma JJ, et al. A clinical trial comparing three antithrombotic-drug regimens after coronary-artery stenting. N Engl J Med 1998;339(23):1665–71.

7. Holmes DR, Reddy VY, Turi ZG, et al. Percutaneous closure of the left atrial appendage versus warfarin therapy for prevention of stroke in patients with atrial fibrillation: a randomised non-inferiority trial. Lancet 2009;374(9689):534–42.

8. Holmes DR, Kar S, Price MJ, et al. Prospective randomized evaluation of the WATCHMAN left atrial appendage closure device in patients with atrial fibrillation versus long-term warfarin therapy: the PREVAIL trial. J Am Coll Cardiol 2014;64(1):1–12.

9. Kirchhof P, Benussi S, Kotecha D, et al. 2016 ESC guidelines for the management of atrial fibrillation developed in collaboration with EACTS. Eur Heart J 2016;37(38):2893–962.

10. Reddy VY, Doshi SK, Kar S, et al. 5-year outcomes after left atrial appendage closure: from the PREVAIL and PROTECT AF trials. J Am Coll Cardiol 2017;70(24):2964–75.

11. Dukkipati SR, Kar S, Holmes DR, et al. Device-related thrombus after left atrial appendage closure: incidence, predictors, and outcomes. Circulation 2018;138(9):874–85.

12. Price MJ, Reddy VY, Valderrábano M, et al. Bleeding outcomes after left atrial appendage closure compared with long-term warfarin a pooled, patient-level analysis of the WATCHMAN randomized trial experience. JACC Cardiovasc Interv 2015;8(15):1925–32.

13. Bergmann MW, Betts TR, Sievert H, et al. Safety and efficacy of early anticoagulation drug regimens after WATCHMAN left atrial appendage closure: three-month data from the EWOLUTION prospective, multicentre, monitored international WATCHMAN LAA closure registry. EuroIntervention 2017;13(7):877–84.

14. Boersma LV, Ince H, Kische S, et al. Evaluating real-world clinical outcomes in atrial fibrillation patients receiving the WATCHMAN left atrial appendage closure technology. Circ Arrhythm Electrophysiol 2019;12(4):e006841.

15. Søndergaard L, Wong YH, Reddy VY, et al. Propensity-matched comparison of oral anticoagulation versus antiplatelet therapy after left atrial appendage closure with WATCHMAN. JACC Cardiovasc Interv 2019;12(11):1055–63.

16. Ketterer U, Giuseppe DA, Siegel I, et al. Percutaneous left atrial appendage occlusion: device thrombosis in clopidogrel non-responders. Resuscitation 2018;81(2):S63.

17. Chun KJ, Bordignon S, Urban V, et al. Left atrial appendage closure followed by 6 weeks of antithrombotic therapy: a prospective single-center experience. Heart Rhythm 2013;10(12):1792–9.

18. Dentali F, Riva N, Crowther M, et al. Efficacy and safety of the novel oral anticoagulants in atrial fibrillation: a systematic review and meta-analysis of the literature. Circulation 2012;126(20):2381–91.

19. Bergmann MW, Betts TR, Sievert H, et al. Early anticoagulation drug regimens after WATCHMAN left atrial appendage closure: safety and efficacy. EuroIntervention 2017;13(7):877–84.

20. Korsholm K, Nielsen KM, Jensen JM, et al. Transcatheter left atrial appendage occlusion in patients with atrial fibrillation and a high bleeding risk using aspirin alone for post-implant antithrombotic therapy. EuroIntervention 2017;12(17):2075–82.

21. Fauchier L, Cinaud A, Brigadeau F, et al. Device-related thrombosis after percutaneous left atrial appendage occlusion for atrial fibrillation. J Am Coll Cardiol 2018;71(14):1528–36.

22. Saw J, Tzikas A, Shakir S, et al. Incidence and clinical impact of device-associated thrombus and peri-device leak following left atrial appendage closure with the Amplatzer cardiac plug. JACC Cardiovasc Interv 2017;10(4):391–9.

23. Lempereur M, Aminian A, Saw J. Device-associated thrombus formation after left atrial appendage occlusion: a systematic review of events reported with the WATCHMAN, the Amplatzer Cardiac Plug and the Amulet. Catheter Cardiovasc Interv 2018;92(3):E210–7.

24. Plicht B, Konorza TFM, Kahlert P, et al. Risk factors for thrombus formation on the Amplatzer cardiac plug after left atrial appendage occlusion. JACC Cardiovasc Interv 2013;6(6):606–13.

25. Shamim S, Magalski A, Chhatriwalla AK, et al. Transesophageal echocardiographic diagnosis of a WATCHMAN left atrial appendage closure device thrombus 10 years following implantation. Echocardiography 2017;34(1):128–30.

26. Mant J, Hobbs R, Fletcher K, et al. Warfarin versus aspirin for stroke prevention in an elderly community population with atrial fibrillation. Results of the BAFTA trial. Lancet 2008;48(2):68.

27. Reddy VY, Möbius-Winkler S, Miller MA, et al. Left atrial appendage closure with the WATCHMAN device in patients with a contraindication for oral

anticoagulation: the ASAP study (ASA Plavix feasibility study with WATCHMAN left atrial appendage closure technology). J Am Coll Cardiol 2013; 61(25):2551–6.

28. Tzikas A, Shakir S, Gafoor S, et al. Left atrial appendage occlusion for stroke prevention in atrial fibrillation: multicenter experience with the ACP. EuroIntervention 2016;11(10):1170–9.

29. Enomoto Y, Gadiyaram VK, Gianni C, et al. Use of non-warfarin oral anticoagulants instead of warfarin during left atrial appendage closure with the WATCHMAN device. Heart Rhythm 2017;14(1): 19–24.

30. Heart IJC, Phillips KP, Santoso T, et al. Left atrial appendage closure with WATCHMAN in Asian patients: 2 year outcomes from the WASP registry. Int J Cardiol Heart Vasc 2019;23:100358.

31. Landmesser U, Tondo C, Camm J, et al. Left atrial appendage occlusion with the AMPLATZER Amulet device: one-year follow-up from the prospective global Amulet observational registry. EuroIntervention 2018;14(5):e590–7.

32. Friberg L, Rosenqvist M, Lip GYH. Evaluation of risk stratification schemes for ischaemic stroke and bleeding in 182 678 patients with atrial fibrillation: the Swedish Atrial Fibrillation cohort study. Eur Heart J 2012;33(12):1500–10.

33. Lip GYH, Frison L, Halperin JL, et al. Comparative validation of a novel risk score for predicting bleeding risk in anticoagulated patients with atrial fibrillation: the HAS-BLED (hypertension, abnormal renal/liver function, stroke, bleeding history or predisposition, labile INR, elderly, drug. J Am Coll Cardiol 2011;57(2):173–80.

Clinical Implications and Management Strategies for Left Atrial Appendage Leaks

Anu Sahore, MD[a], Domenico G. Della Rocca, MD[a,*],
Alisara Anannab, MD[a,b], Sanghamitra Mohanty, MD[a], Krishna Akella, DO[c],
Ghulam Murtaza, MD[c], Chintan Trivedi, MD, MPH[a], Carola Gianni, MD, PhD[a],
Qiong Chen, MD[a], Mohamed Bassiouny, MD[a],
Ashkan Ahmadian-Tehrani, MD[d], Bryan Macdonald, MD[a],
Amin Al-Ahmad, MD[a], Nicola Tarantino, MD[e], Donatello Cirone, MPH[f],
Rodney P. Horton, MD[a], Jorge Romero, MD[e], Dhanunjaya Lakkireddy, MD[c],
Luigi Di Biase, MD, PhD[a,e,g,h,i], Andrea Natale, MD[a,g,h,i,j,k,l]

KEYWORDS

- Leak • Left atrial appendage • Stroke • Watchman • Lariat • Outcome • Amulet
- Transient ischemic attach

KEY POINTS

- There is significant variation of reported leak rates following left atrial appendage (LAA) closure procedures.
- Leaks resulting from incomplete surgical ligation of LAA have been associated with an increased risk of thromboembolic (TE) events.
- It is still debated whether a correlation between TE events and leaks resulting from percutaneous procedures exists.
- It is current clinical practice to continue oral anticoagulation (OAC) in presence of a significant peri-device leak, if clinically feasible.

INTRODUCTION

Left atrial appendage (LAA) is well known as the dominant source of thrombus formation in patients with nonvalvular atrial fibrillation (AF)[1,2]. For years, oral anticoagulation (OAC) has been the standard of care for stroke prophylaxis in patients with a diagnosis of AF. However, OAC may significantly increase the risk of bleeding events, especially in the presence of specific comorbidities and risk factors (eg, liver disease, chronic kidney disease, and recurrent falls).[3,4] In view of these factors,

[a] Texas Cardiac Arrhythmia Institute, St. David's Medical Center, Austin, TX, USA; [b] Department of Cardiovascular Intervention, Central Chest Institute of Thailand, Nonthaburi, Thailand; [c] Kansas City Heart Rhythm Institute & Research Foundation, Overland Park, KS, USA; [d] Department of Medicine, Division of Internal Medicine, University of Texas Health Science Center, San Antonio, TX, USA; [e] Arrhythmia Services, Department of Medicine, Montefiore Medical Center, Albert Einstein College of Medicine, Bronx, NY, USA; [f] Azienda Ospedaliero-Universitaria Careggi, Florence, Italy; [g] Department of Internal Medicine, Dell Medical School, University of Texas, Austin, TX, USA; [h] Department of Biomedical Engineering, Cockrell School of Engineering, University of Texas, Austin, TX, USA; [i] Department of Clinical and Experimental Medicine, University of Foggia, Foggia, Italy; [j] Interventional Electrophysiology, Scripps Clinic, La Jolla, CA, USA; [k] Department of Cardiology, Metro-Health Medical Center, Case Western Reserve University School of Medicine, Cleveland, OH, USA; [l] Division of Cardiology, Stanford University, Stanford, CA, USA
* Corresponding author. Texas Cardiac Arrhythmia Institute, St. David's Medical Center, 3000 North I-35, Suite 720, Austin, TX 78705.
E-mail address: domenicodellarocca@hotmail.it

Card Electrophysiol Clin 12 (2020) 89–96
https://doi.org/10.1016/j.ccep.2019.11.010
1877-9182/20/© 2019 Elsevier Inc. All rights reserved.

various strategies to exclude the LAA from systemic circulation have been developed over the years, ranging from surgical ligation to percutaneous closure devices.[5–9]

Nevertheless, some patients can display incomplete LAA closure.[10,11] Leaks can result from a suboptimal procedure, or develop during follow-up because of tissue remodeling.[12] In addition, some LAA anatomic features are associated with a higher likelihood of suboptimal LAA exclusion.[13] Resulting leaks can increase or decrease in size overtime.

The aim of this article is to evaluate the clinical implications of incomplete LAA closure, as well as report current and potential upcoming strategies to manage LAA leaks.

CLINICAL CONSIDERATIONS

LAA is derived from the primordial left atrium and is formed by absorption of primordial pulmonary veins and their branches.[14,15] In a normally functioning heart, LAA has intact contractility and blood flow.[2] In patients with AF, LAA can act as a static pouch for blood stagnation because of impaired contractility and ineffective blood flow, thus predisposing to thrombus formation.[2] However, some studies have reported up to 5% of patients who demonstrated LAA thrombi despite being in sinus rhythm.[16] These observations suggest that LAA may potentially serve as a source of atrial thrombi even in absence of AF.

Ischemic stroke and TE events are the major cause of morbidity among patients with AF.[1] Thus, stroke prevention is a critical component of AF management. For more than 60 years, vitamin K antagonists (VKAs) have been the standard of care for TE prophylaxis in patients with AF.[17] However, factors such as continuous monitoring, dietary restrictions, bleeding predisposition may contribute to compliance issues.

In recent years, novel oral anticoagulation agents (NOACs) have been proven to be noninferior in efficacy and somehow superior in terms of safety. Studies, such as ROCKET AF and ARISTOTLE, have shown a lower incidence of intracranial and fatal bleeding events compared with VKA.[18,19] Optimal plan of TE prophylaxis is a fine balance between benefits (TE prevention) and risks (bleeding events). As reported, adherence to NOACs is still poor, even though they do not require continuous monitoring, have a better safety profile, and display fewer drug-drug or drug-food interactions compared with warfarin. As a result, up to 40% of patients with AF still do not receive appropriate anticoagulation due to either poor compliance or presence of contraindications to these agents, despite a high risk of stroke.[20]

To fill this therapeutic gap, various nonpharmacological strategies have been proposed for LAA exclusion, especially in patients who cannot tolerate long-term OAC. LAA exclusion can be achieved with surgical suturing, hybrid, or nonsurgical percutaneous device placement methods. Various major trials have supported the concept that excluding the LAA from systemic circulation effectively decreases the incidence of cerebrovascular events.[5–9]

The 2019 AHA/ACC/HRS Focused Update of the 2014 AHA/ACC/HRS Guideline for the Management of Patients With Atrial Fibrillation[21] recommends considering:

1. Surgical occlusion of the LAA in patients with AF and high risk of stroke undergoing cardiac surgery (recommendation class IIb, level of evidence: B).
2. Percutaneous LAA occlusion for stroke prevention in patients with AF with a high risk of stroke who have contraindications to long-term anticoagulation (recommendation class IIb, level of evidence: B).

However, as per Centers of Medicare and Medicaid Services, LAA occlusion devices may only be considered in patients in whom long-term OAC is contraindicated and have a CHADS2 score ≥ 2 or a CHA2DS2-VASc score ≥ 3.

Because of the technique used for LAA exclusion, antithrombotic treatment may be required to prevent device-related thrombosis. This complication may occur in cases of endocardial LAA closure procedures until adequate endothelialization of the device is achieved. Conversely, incomplete LAA occlusion may result from any of the above-mentioned LAA exclusion techniques (specifically surgical, hybrid, percutaneous) thereby potentially hampering an effective TE prophylaxis. Thus, it is of utmost importance to understand the incidence and natural history of residual leaks following LAA closure procedures, as well as their impact on clinical outcomes.

MAJOR TECHNIQUES OF LEFT ATRIAL APPENDAGE EXCLUSION
Epicardial Approach

Surgical ligation
Postoperative AF is highly prevalent (2%−7%) and is associated with a significant risk of stroke especially in patients with coronary bypass surgery.[22] Current practice and guidelines recommend surgical closure of LAA in patients with AF undergoing mitral valve, Maze, and coronary artery bypass graft surgeries.[21] Surgical LAA exclusion is usually

performed during open heart surgery while the heart is on a heart-lung pump. Cardiac chambers are empty and myocardium is flaccid during the procedure. Therefore, placing a self-retaining knot around the neck of the appendage can be as difficult as tying a rubber band around a deflated balloon.[12,23] Thus, surgical exclusion of LAA can often yield incomplete closure. Incomplete closure of LAA postsurgical exclusion methods (excision, suture, slip, or stapler exclusion) has been reported to be up to 60% (Table 1).[23]

Residual flow between the left atrial cavity and the postsurgical remnant of the LAA can be classified as:

1. Incompletely surgically ligated LAA (ISLL): ISLL is referred to as the presence of a narrow, constricted LAA neck connecting the intact LAA to the left atrial cavity.
2. LAA stump: It is defined by the presence of a short LAA vestige measuring ≥ 1.0 cm in depth.

Hybrid approach
LAA exclusion via the Lariat device (SentreHeart, Redwood City, CA) consists of a pretied suture loop guided by an endocardial magnetic-tipped wire delivered over the LAA. The device comprises 3 components: a complaint occlusion balloon catheter, 0.025- and 0.035-inch magnet-tipped guidewires, and a 12-F suture delivery device. Preprocedural transesophageal echocardiography (TEE) is performed to rule out LAA thrombus under anesthesia. Epicardial access and transseptal access for endocardial guidewire are first established. An endocardial magnet-tipped guidewire is then placed at the apex of the LAA with balloon identification of LAA ostium. The epicardial and endocardial magnet-tipped guidewires work as a rail used to snare capture of LAA and release the pretied suture for appendage ligation.

Lariat is contraindicated in patients with a history of pericarditis or cardiac surgery, recent myocardial infarction in the last 3 months, and chest wall abnormalities, such as pectus excavatum, history of thoracic radiation exposure. Various LAA-related contraindications are (1) LAA width greater than 40 mm; (2) superiorly located LAA with LAA apex directed behind the pulmonary trunk; (3) bilobed LAA or multilobed LAA in which lobes are oriented in different planes exceeding 40 mm; (4) posteriorly rotated heart; and (5) LAA thrombus detected on preprocedural TEE.[8]

Table 1
Incidence of incomplete left atrial appendage closure

LAA Occlusion Technique	Study	Study Design	Reported Leak Rate, %	Imaging Modality Used	Imaging Follow-Up
Surgical ligation	Aryana et al,[32] 2015	Nonrandomized prospective	24	CT angiography	3 mo
	Kanderian et al,[23] 2008	Retrospective	34	TEE	8.1 ± 12 mo
Watchman device	Holmes et al,[6] 2014	Prospective randomized	32	TEE	45 d–2 y
	Pillarisetti et al,[10] 2013	Multicenter prospective observational	21	TEE	1 y
	Cochet et al,[31] 2018	Prospective observational	44	CT (Arterial phase)	>3 mo
LARIAT	Bartus et al,[7] 2013	Nonrandomized single center	5	TEE	30–90 d
	Lakkireddy et al,[8] 2016	Prospective observational	13	TEE	30–90 d
	Pillarisetti et al,[10] 2015	Multicenter prospective observational	14	TEE	1 y
Amulet/ACP	Landmesser et al,[30] 2017	Multicenter prospective observational	1.8	TEE	67 ± 23 d
	Cochet et al,[31] 2018	Prospective observational	43	CT (arterial phase)	>3 mo
			72	CT (venous phase)	

The acute procedural success rate ranges between 94% and 98%.[7,8,24] Leaks resulting from a Lariat device placement are centrally located, similarly to those from surgical ligation procedures. As the suture ties down the neck of the LAA, a central leak can develop (so-called gunny sack effect).[10,12] Incidence of leaks ranges between 0% and 26%[10,12,25,26] and depends on several factors, including operators' experience, site of suture application, and the imaging technique used for follow-up (See **Table 1**).

On a pathophysiological standpoint, leaks are classified as:

- Acute leaks, developed at the time of procedure, as a result of suboptimal tightening of the suture. Those leaks might close overtime, owing to endothelialization or fibrosis.
- Early (within 6 months) or late (after 6 months) leaks, are related to knot slippage, owing to tissue necrosis or suboptimal tightening. If the suture loop is created too close to the left atrium, atrial tissue may bunch up at the neck, which can potentially unfurl and create a central leak. The tissue inside the loop gets remodeled over time and can result in communication between the atrial cavity and remnant LAA cavity. Those leaks are less likely to close over time.

Other factors contributing to leak formation are:

- Misalignment of the suture or the magnets, which may jeopardize an effective suture tensuring and placement.
- Multi-lobar anatomy of the LAA, potentially resulting in selective ligation of one lobe, leaving the others patent.

Percutaneous Approach

There are several endocardial LAA closure devices available. Among them, the Watchman device (Boston Scientific, Natick, MA), the Amplatzer cardiac plug (ACP; St. Jude Medical, Minneapolis, MN), and the Amulet device (St. Jude Medical) are the most commonly used.

The Watchman device (Boston Scientific) is a parachute-shaped, self-expanding nitinol frame structure with 12 active fixation barbs radially distributed to anchor the device to the LAA walls.[5,6] Its atrium-facing side is covered with a permeable polyester membrane that acts as a filter to capture emboli that might be developed in the LAA cavity. In addition, the membrane promotes endothelialization over the device. It is deployed after transseptal puncture via a percutaneous catheter-based delivery system.

The Watchman device is manufactured in 5 different sizes, ranging from 21 to 33 mm (3 mm increments). Selected size is generally 10% to 20% larger than the largest size of LAA ostium to ensure stability and prevent dislodgment. It has been demonstrated to be noninferior to warfarin for stroke prevention in patients with AF in PROTECT-AF and PREVAIL trials.[5,6] The more recent EWOLUTION registry[27] (Registry on Watchman Outcomes in Real-Life Utilization) involving 1025 patients, showed better procedural success rate and safety profile compared with those reported in the PROTECT-AF and PREVAIL trials. These observations suggest improvement in implant techniques, with better operator training over the years. Overall, the reported success rate of Watchman implantation ranges between 91% and 98.5%.[5,6,12,27]

The AMPLATZER Cardiac Plug[9,13,28] (ACP; St. Jude Medical, Maple Grove, MN) is a self-expanding device and consists of a lobe and a disk connected with a central articulated waist. The lobe and disk face the LAA cavity and the LA side, respectively. The lobe has fixation wires for device stabilization. The proximal disk is intended to cover the LAA ostium and is 4 to 6 mm larger in diameter than the distal lobe.

The Amplatzer Amulet device (St. Jude Medical, Maple Grove, MN) is the second generation of ACP. It has a similar disk and lobe structure and is available in 8 different sizes ranging from 11 to 31 mm. Compared with the ACP, whose difference in diameter between disk and lobe was 4 to 6 mm, the proximal disk of the Amulet is 6 to 7 mm larger than the proximal lobe.

The reported success rate of ACP and Amulet ranges from 94.6% to 100%.[9,29,30]

LAA is a complex geometric structure with oval orifice. It has an elliptical morphology and available endocardial devices are circular in shape. This can cause incomplete sealing at the periphery of the device and the atrial wall, also known as "edge effect."[12] Even if complete LAA sealing is achieved immediately by selecting a larger device to get good compression and stability, eventual tissue remodeling can contribute to peridevice leak formation.

Other factors associated with incomplete LAA closure are LA dilation, non-chicken wing LAA shape, large landing zone size, and misalignment of disk and lobe (in ACP and Amulet).[29]

Reported incidence of leaks is 15% to 44% for the Watchman[10,11,31] and 1.8% to 43% for the ACP/Amulet devices (See **Table 1**).[9,10,29]

CLINICAL IMPLICATIONS

Incomplete LAA exclusion procedures lead to a persistent communication between LAA cavity and systemic circulation. As a result, a thrombus forming inside the LAA can still be a potential source of emboli. Whether small leaks are associated with an increased TE risk is still a matter of debate. It is common practice not to interrupt OAC in patients with leaks greater than 5 mm in size. However, this 5-mm threshold has been nonuniform and completely arbitrary, because the available literature inconsistently correlated larger leaks with a higher incidence of stroke.[11,26,29,32]

Leaks After Surgical Exclusion

ISLL was associated with a significantly higher incidence of TE events. Specifically, Aryana and colleagues[32] reported an annualized risk of TE events per 100 patient-years of 6.5% for ISLL patients, compared with a 1.9% risk for the entire study group. The incidence of TE events was even higher in those ISLL patients with a residual neck diameter of less than 5 mm (19.0% per 100 patient-years).

Leaks After Hybrid LAA Procedures

In a series of 98 patients who received the Lariat,[25] 5 (5.1%) neurologic TE events (4 strokes and 1 transient ischemic attack [TIA]) were documented during a follow-up of 16 ± 2.5 months. Of these, 3 occurred after 6 months of follow-up, all being associated with small (<5 mm) leaks.

Similar observations were noted in a larger series of 306 patients who received the Lariat.[26] At 4-week TEE follow-up, leaks were documented in 26.5% of patients and all were less than 5 mm. Over a follow-up period of 15.9 ± 9.2 months, 9 (2.9%) TE events were reported, 7 occurring in patients with a documented leak. Incidence of TE events was significantly higher among patients with a persistent leak (11.7% [7/60] vs 0.81% [2/246]; P<.001). As previously mentioned, all events occurred with leaks less than 5 mm.

Leaks After Endocardial LAA Closure

Existing literature has not yet demonstrated a significant correlation between incomplete LAA occlusion and increased risk of TE events, regardless of the endocardial device used to close the appendage.[11,29] In a substudy of the PROTECT-AF,[11] follow-up TEE revealed at least some degree of peridevice residual flow in 32% of patients with successful Watchman implantation.

The severity of flow was minor in 7.7% of patients with residual flow, and moderate and major in 59.9% and 32.4%, respectively. The average and maximum leak width was 2.9 and 6 mm at 12 months postimplant. No statistical relationship was documented between the presence and size of leak and a composite embolic endpoint of stroke and systemic embolization. In a comparative study by Pillarisetti and colleagues,[10] patients who received the Watchman had a significantly higher incidence of leaks at 12 months compared with those who received the Lariat (21% vs 13%, P = .019). In addition, post-Watchman leaks were wider than post-Lariat ones (3.10 ± 1.1 vs 2.15 ± 1.4 mm; P = .001). TE events were documented in 3 out of 219 patients in the Watchman group, 2 of them occurring in patients without documented residual peridevice flow.

A lack of correlation between residual peridevice flow and occurrence of TE events was similarly observed in patients who received the ACP and Amulet.[29] In a recent study by Saw and colleagues,[29] presence of peridevice leak was assessed in 311 patients after successful ACP implantation. Complete LAA closure was documented in 80.2% of patients, whereas residual leaks were graded as minimal (<1 mm) in 5.5% patients, mild (1–3 mm) in 5.8%, moderate (4–5 mm) in 0.6%, and severe (>5 mm) in 0.6%. Residual LAA flow was not associated with an increased risk of cardiovascular events (stroke, TIA, cardiovascular death, overall mortality). In univariate and multivariate analysis, no independent predictors of cardiovascular events were identified.

Several factors might explain this lack of evidence between peridevice leaks and TE events in patients with endovascular devices compared with those with a previous hybrid and surgical LAA closure. First, the observed incidence of TE events is consistently low in all studies enrolling patients undergoing percutaneous LAA occlusion. As a result, the relatively limited sample size might have contributed to the lack of statistical significance between leaks and clinical outcomes. Second, 2D-TEE has been routinely used to quantify the presence of residual flow during follow-up. However, the risk of misclassification and undersizing of peridevice leaks has been demonstrated to be significantly higher with this imaging technique[31] compared with 3D-TEE or computed tomography (CT).

Leaks can be detected with various available imaging modalities at the time of procedure or during the follow-up period. Intraprocedural TEE and fluoroscopy with contrast medium injection are used to assess for incomplete closure.

Multiple views are required for accurate assessment of LAA sealing and device position. With 2D-TEE a complete assessment of the edges of an endovascular device, as well as an adequate view of the surface of the ligated LAA walls facing the LA, can be challenging. As a result, the diagnostic yield of this technique in identifying residual leaks is limited.

3D-TEE has been shown to be more accurate than 2D-TEE for visualization and quantitative analysis of the LAA orifice; its findings are comparable with those from multislice CT.[25] A possible explanation for the inconsistency of leak prevalence between studies might be related to the different imaging techniques adopted to assess them. As a matter of fact, studies using CT or 3D-TEE have reported higher rate of LAA leaks.[25,31]

Unlike TEE, CT does not require direct visualization of the leak jet detection. LAA patency is demonstrated by contrast uptake related to the presence of leaks; those leaks are sometimes inaccessible to TEE, specifically submillimetric marginal leaks, transfabric leaks, and small defects of endothelialization.

Earlier data have also documented a significant difference of maximal LAA width measurements between CT and TEE (CT 25.8 ± 4.7 mm; TEE 25.1 ± 4.4 mm; $P = .016$).[33] This can potentially affect the accuracy of device size selection, thereby increasing the risk of incomplete LAA closure.

MANAGEMENT STRATEGIES IN THE PRESENCE OF PERIDEVICE LEAK

It is current practice not to discontinue OAC if a leak greater than 5 mm is documented, regardless of the procedure adopted for LAA closure. However, as mentioned above, an increased risk of TE events has been documented in patients with persistent LAA patency resulting from surgical ligation and Lariat procedures[26,32]; this risk seems to be independent from leak severity. Therefore, continuation of OAC is recommended in these patients. In patients with incomplete percutaneous LAA closure procedures due to a moderate leak (3–5 mm), it is reasonable to consider other factors when deciding whether OAC should be continued. In addition to some patient-related factors (eg, history of recurrent TE events, high CHA_2DS_2-VASc score), it is our common practice to individualize our strategy based on certain clinical and anatomic considerations. Among them, left atrial dense spontaneous echo-contrast (LASEC) is due to an interaction between red cells and plasma proteins, and is independent from platelet

activation. LASEC is an epiphenomenon of cardiac conditions (eg, valvulopathies, atrial arrhythmias) that promotes atrial enlargement and blood stasis. Given this hypercoagulable state, it might be reasonable not to discontinue OAC even in the presence of moderate (3–5 mm) leaks.

Other factors that should be considered in patients with a documented leak is the presence and size of a thrombus within the LAA after closure. In our experience, the morphology of a thrombus formed inside the LAA can be used as supplemental evidence to assess the significance of peridevice leaks on TEE. Specifically, incomplete thrombus formation or absence of evident thrombi seem to indicate a significant residual peridevice flow irrespective of the leak size documented by 2D-TEE.

Although the clinical impact of LASEC and thrombus morphology in the setting of incomplete LAA closure has not been assessed yet, it is prudent to consider these and other clinical, anatomic, and imaging features when deciding whether or not to stop OAC in cases of borderline (3–5 mm) leaks.

Use of Percutaneous Devices for Leak Closure

Various exclusion and occlusion devices and techniques have developed for closure of LAA leaks. Concentric leaks after applying a Lariat device can be closed using an Amplatzer septal occluder (ASO) device or by repeat Lariat application.[34] The ASO device was originally designed for atrial septal defect closure and has been used for closure of LAA leaks.

Even if there are few reported cases of successful closure of leaks after percutaneous devices using ASO, those leaks created might be difficult to approach given the eccentric jets from the leaks.

In these patients, endovascular coils have been tested in a single-center prospective trial (TREASURE), which reported closure of both eccentric and central residual leaks in 30 patients.

In a recent report, the Watchman device was used in 7 patients with chronically failed closure after surgical ligation. Successful closure of leak was achieved even with narrow neck (≤10 mm) of ISLL with requirement of poststenotic dilation of the remnant of LAA body.[35] This included patients who received internal ligation, stapled excision, or surgical excision.

SUMMARY

Incomplete LAA closure is a common finding following surgical, hybrid, and percutaneous procedures for LAA exclusion. Although a clear correlation between persistent LAA patency and risk of

TE events has not been consistently confirmed, it is reasonable to continue OAC in all patients with a residual leak greater than 5 mm. Whether patients with a moderate (3–5 mm) leak should be considered at risk for TE events, it is still a matter of debate. An individualized approach based on certain clinical and anatomic features should be considered in these patients. However, further studies are needed to elucidate the clinical impact of these factors and their value for stratification of TE risk in patients with incomplete LAA closure. As an alternative to OAC, several device-based strategies for leak closure have been tested in small studies. Additional work is necessary to assess their safety and effectiveness.

REFERENCES

1. Williams BA, Honushefsky AM, Berger PB. Temporal trends in the incidence, prevalence, and survival of patients with atrial fibrillation from 2004 to 2016. Am J Cardiol 2017;120:1961–5.
2. Stoddard MF, Dawkins PR, Prince CR, et al. Left atrial appendage thrombus is not uncommon in patients with acute atrial fibrillation and a recent embolic event: a transesophageal echocardiographics tudy. J Am Coll Cardiol 1995;25:452–9.
3. Gadiyaram VK, Mohanty S, Gianni C, et al. Thromboembolic events and need for anticoagulation therapy following left atrial appendage occlusion in patients with electrical isolation of the appendage. J Cardiovasc Electrophysiol 2019;30:511–6.
4. Kakkar AK, Mueller I, Bassand J-P, et al. Risk profiles and antithrombotic treatment of patients newly diagnosed with atrial fibrillation at risk of stroke: perspectives from the international, observational, prospective GARFIELD registry. Hernandez AV, ed. PLoS One 2013;8:e63479.
5. Reddy VY, Sievert H, Halperin J, et al. Percutaneous left atrial appendage closure vs warfarin for atrial fibrillation: a randomized clinical trial. JAMA 2014; 312:1988.
6. Holmes DR, Kar S, Price MJ, et al. Prospective randomized evaluation of the watchman left atrial appendage closure device in patients with atrial fibrillation versus long-term warfarin therapy. J Am Coll Cardiol 2014;64:1–12.
7. Bartus K, Han FT, Bednarek J, et al. Percutaneous left atrial appendage suture ligation using the LARIAT device in patients with atrial fibrillation. J Am Coll Cardiol 2013;62:108–18.
8. Lakkireddy D, Afzal MR, Lee RJ, et al. Short and long-term outcomes of percutaneous left atrial appendage suture ligation: results from a US multicenter evaluation. Heart Rhythm 2016;13:1030–6.
9. Tzikas A, Shakir S, Gafoor S, et al. Left atrial appendage occlusion for stroke prevention in atrial fibrillation: multicentre experience with the AMPLATZER cardiac plug. EuroIntervention 2016;11:1170–9.
10. Pillarisetti J, Reddy YM, Gunda S, et al. Endocardial (Watchman) vs epicardial (Lariat) left atrial appendage exclusion devices: understanding the differences in the location and type of leaks and their clinical implications. Heart Rhythm 2015;12: 1501–7.
11. Viles-Gonzalez JF, Kar S, Douglas P, et al. The clinical impact of incomplete left atrial appendage closure with the watchman device in patients with atrial fibrillation. J Am Coll Cardiol 2012;59:923–9.
12. Yarlagadda B, Parikh V, Dar T, et al. Leaks after left atrial appendage ligation with Lariat device: incidence, pathophysiology, clinical implications and methods of closure—a case based discussion. J Atr Fibrillation 2017;10:1725.
13. Saw J, Fahmy P, Spencer R, et al. Comparing measurements of CT angiography, TEE, and fluoroscopy of the left atrial appendage for percutaneous closure: comparing measurements of CT angiography, TEE, and fluoroscopy. J Cardiovasc Electrophysiol 2016;27:414–22.
14. Della Rocca DG, Mohanty S, Trivedi C, et al. Percutaneous treatment of non-paroxysmal atrial fibrillation: a paradigm shift from pulmonary vein to nonpulmonary vein trigger ablation? Arrhythm Electrophysiol Rev 2018;7:256.
15. Di Biase L, Romero J, Briceno D, et al. Evidence of relevant electrical connection between the left atrial appendage and the great cardiac vein during catheter ablation of atrial fibrillation. Heart Rhythm 2019; 16:1039–46.
16. Labovitz AJ. Transesophageal echocardiography and unexplained cerebral ischemia: a multicenter follow-up study. Am Heart J 1999;137:1082–7.
17. Birman-Deych E, Radford MJ, Nilasena DS, et al. Use and effectiveness of warfarin in medicare beneficiaries with atrial fibrillation. Stroke 2006;37: 1070–4.
18. Patel MR, Mahaffey KW, Garg J, et al. Rivaroxaban versus warfarin in nonvalvular atrial fibrillation. N Engl J Med 2011;365:883–91.
19. Granger CB, Alexander JH, McMurray JJV, et al. Apixaban versus warfarin in patients with atrial fibrillation. N Engl J Med 2011;365:981–92.
20. Go AS, Hylek EM, Phillips KA, et al. Prevalence of diagnosed atrial fibrillation in adults: national implications for rhythm management and stroke prevention: the AnTicoagulation and Risk Factors in Atrial Fibrillation (ATRIA) study. JAMA 2001;285:2370.
21. January CT, Wann LS, Calkins H, et al. 2019 AHA/ACC/HRS focused update of the 2014 AHA/ACC/HRS guideline for the management of patients with atrial fibrillation: a report of the American College of Cardiology/American Heart Association Task Force on Clinical Practice Guidelines and the Heart

Rhythm Society in Collaboration with the Society of Thoracic Surgeons. Heart Rhythm 2019;16:e66–93. Available at: https://www.ahajournals.org/doi/10.1161/CIR.0000000000000665. Accessed September 9, 2019.

22. Damiano RJ, Gaynor SL, Bailey M, et al. The long-term outcome of patients with coronary disease and atrial fibrillation undergoing the cox maze procedure. J Thorac Cardiovasc Surg 2003;126: 2016–21.

23. Kanderian AS, Gillinov AM, Pettersson GB, et al. Success of surgical left atrial appendage closure. J Am Coll Cardiol 2008;52:924–9.

24. Price MJ, Gibson DN, Yakubov SJ, et al. Early safety and efficacy of percutaneous left atrial appendage suture ligation. J Am Coll Cardiol 2014;64:565–72.

25. Gianni C, Di Biase L, Trivedi C, et al. Clinical implications of leaks following left atrial appendage ligation with the LARIAT device. JACC Cardiovasc Interv 2016;9:1051–7.

26. Mohanty S, Gianni C, Trivedi C, et al. Risk of thromboembolic events after percutaneous left atrial appendage ligation in patients with atrial fibrillation: long-term results from a multicenter study. Heart Rhythm 2019. https://doi.org/10.1016/j.hrthm.2019.08.003.

27. Boersma LV, Ince H, Kische S, et al. Efficacy and safety of left atrial appendage closure with WATCHMAN in patients with or without contraindication to oral anticoagulation: 1-year follow-up outcome data of the EWOLUTION trial. Heart Rhythm 2017;14:1302–8.

28. Kar S, Hou D, Jones R, et al. Impact of Watchman and Amplatzer devices on left atrial appendage adjacent structures and healing response in a canine model. JACC Cardiovasc Interv 2014;7: 801–9.

29. Saw J, Tzikas A, Shakir S, et al. Incidence and clinical impact of device-associated thrombus and peri-device leak following left atrial appendage closure with the Amplatzer cardiac plug. JACC Cardiovasc Interv 2017;10:391–9.

30. Landmesser U, Schmidt B, Nielsen-Kudsk JE, et al. Left atrial appendage occlusion with the AMPLATZER Amulet device: periprocedural and early clinical/echocardiographic data from a global prospective observational study. EuroIntervention 2017;13:867–76.

31. Cochet H, Iriart X, Sridi S, et al. Left atrial appendage patency and device-related thrombus after percutaneous left atrial appendage occlusion: a computed tomography study. Eur Heart J Cardiovasc Imaging 2018;19:1351–61.

32. Aryana A, Singh SK, Singh SM, et al. Association between incomplete surgical ligation of left atrial appendage and stroke and systemic embolization. Heart Rhythm 2015;12:1431–7.

33. Wang DD, Eng M, Kupsky D, et al. Application of 3-dimensional computed tomographic image guidance to WATCHMAN implantation and impact on early operator learning curve. JACC Cardiovasc Interv 2016;9:2329–40.

34. Pillai AM, Kanmanthareddy A, Earnest M, et al. Initial experience with post Lariat left atrial appendage leak closure with Amplatzer septal occluder device and repeat Lariat application. Heart Rhythm 2014; 11:1877–83.

35. Ellis CR, Metawee M, Piana RN, et al. Feasibility of left atrial appendage device closure following chronically failed surgical ligation. Heart Rhythm 2019;16: 12–7.

Epicardial versus Endocardial Closure
Is One Better than the Other?

Krishna Akella, DO[a], Bharath Yarlagadda, MD[b], Ghulam Murtaza, MD[a],
Domenico G. Della Rocca, MD[c,d], Rakesh Gopinathannair, MD, FHRS[a],
Andrea Natale, MD, FHRS[c,d], Dhanunjaya Lakkireddy, MD, FHRS[a,*]

KEYWORDS

• Left atrial appendage occlusion • Epicardial • Endocardial

KEY POINTS

• Left Atrial Appendage occlusion devices are a rapidly emerging technology geared towards stroke risk reduction in patients with rationale to discontinue anticoagulation.
• Although devices appear to have similar outcome profile, more trials are performed on each emerging device will help clarify the differences between epicardial and endocardial devices.
• Clear physiologic difference between epicardial and endocardial approach but ideal candidates are different
• Epicardial and endocardial approaches demonstrate clear differences in measured biomarkers. The long term clinical implication and determination of ideal candidates for each device is yet to be determined.
• As this technology develops, differences among devices will yield better outcomes in future generations of devices and management strategy geared towards prevention of complications.

INTRODUCTION

Thrombus in the left atrial appendage (LAA) contributes to 90% of atrial fibrillation (AF) -related strokes.[1] Whether it is the result of low flow state, the presence of scar tissue, or systemic hypercoagulability, the LAA is predisposed toward the formation of thromboembolism.[2–5] Oral anticoagulation has been shown to reduce the incidence of stroke by up to 64%. Currently, anticoagulation with warfarin or direct oral anticoagulants (DOACs) is used for stroke prophylaxis in AF patients with CHADS-VaSC (composite score comprised of Congestive heart failure, Hypertension, Age greater than 65/75, Diabetes mellitus, Stroke history, Vascular disease history, and female Sex Category) of greater than 2. There is a large proportion of patients who are not candidates for anticoagulation (high bleeding risk, high risk for medication interaction, or noncompliant with their medication, because of inconvenience, bleeding, or cost). Left atrial appendage occlusion (LAAO) with epicardial or endocardial techniques shows promise in these patients. Early randomized controlled trials (RCT) have shown that LAAO is noninferior to warfarin in terms of stroke prophylaxis.

Although originally considered to be an embryologic vestige of the primitive atrium, a greater

[a] The Kansas City heart rhythm institution and research foundation, HCA MIDWEST HEALTH, Second Floor, 5100 W 110th St, Overland Park, KS 66211, USA; [b] Department of Cardiology, University of New Mexico, 1 University of New Mexico, Albuquerque, NM 87131, USA; [c] Texas Cardiac Arrhythmia Institute, Center for Atrial Fibrillation at St. David's Medical Center, 1015 East 32nd Street, Suite 516, Austin, TX 78705, USA; [d] Department of Biomedical Engineering, University of Texas, 107 West Dean Keeton Street, Austin, TX 78712, USA
* Corresponding author.
E-mail address: dlakkireddy@kchri.org

1877-9182/20/© 2019 Elsevier Inc. All rights reserved.

understanding of the role the LAA plays in normal physiology and pathology is emerging. Aside from neurohormonal modulation via atrial natriuretic peptide (ANP) production and a possible relationship to renin-angiotensin-aldosterone system (RAAS) regulation, the LAA serves a mechanical function as a decompression chamber and contractile reserve for the left atrium.[6–9] LAAO has the potential to affect systemic homeostasis favorably because of the aforementioned ANP/RAAS modulation. Moreover, the LAA also plays a role in the development and maintenance of arrhythmia. In 2% to 27% of patients with recurrent AF after ablation, the LAA is responsible for maintenance of the circuit or focus for atrial tachycardia. LAA closure with resultant electrical isolation in addition to AF ablation demonstrated better outcomes when compared with ablation alone.[10,11]

There are 2 main percutaneous approaches to LAAO: epicardial exclusion by suture ligation and endocardial occlusion with a mechanical barrier (**Fig. 1**). Both approaches have their own advantages and limitations. In this review, the authors aim to discuss the differences in techniques, safety, efficacy, and complication profiles of epicardial and endocardial closure devices.

Indications and Contraindications

The most commonly studied LAAO systems in the United States include the LARIAT (AtriCure, Inc., Mason, OH) (epicardial exclusion), WATCHMAN (Boston Scientific, Inc., Marlborough, MA), AMPLATZER Cardiac Plug (ACP) (Abbott, St Paul, MN), and Amulet Abbott, St Paul, MN) (the latter three are endocardial occlusion devices). The ACP is the first iteration of a dedicated LAA closure device. The ACP was superseded by the Amulet device, which is a second-generation closure device. For the purposes of this topic, only the Amulet device is discussed. WATCHMAN is currently the only Food and Drug Administration (FDA) -approved device for LAAO. WATCHMAN is indicated for patients with high CHA2DS2-VASc

who are suitable for short-term warfarin use and who have a rationale to pursue a nonpharmacologic alternative to warfarin. Contraindications include presence of thrombus on echocardiogram, presence of atrial septal defect, patent foramen ovale or closure device, unsuitable anatomy, not candidates for percutaneous catheterization (small patient size, active infection, or bleeding disorder), cannot tolerate aspirin, warfarin, or clopidogrel, and hypersensitivity to device material. Unlike WATCHMAN, Amulet and LARIAT are used off label for LAAO. LARIAT has FDA clearance for soft tissue ligation and provides the added benefit of arrhythmia modulation (discussed further in later discussion). Similar to endocardial devices, LARIAT is contraindicated with the presence of intracardiac thrombus. The presence of adhesions can obstruct the ability of the snare to advance over the LAA; hence, conditions whereby adhesions may be present because of prior insult, such as prior pericarditis, thoracic radiation, or prior pericardiotomy, are considered contraindications in addition to anatomic exclusions listed in later discussion.

Anatomic Considerations and Preprocedural Evaluation

Patients are screened for candidacy using transesophageal echocardiography and/or cardiac computed tomography (CT). To accommodate the WATCHMAN device, the maximum LAA ostium size should be ≥17 and ≤31 mm. In addition, because of its shape, it requires enough depth to be well seated. Similar to the WATCHMAN device, the optimum LAA ostium size accommodating the second-generation Amulet device should be ≥17 mm and ≤32 mm. In contrast to WATCHMAN, the Amulet system can be used for shallower appendages. Other anatomic considerations for endocardial occlusion devices include the shape of the LAA (sharp angles with chicken-wing morphology, short neck less than 10 mm with cauliflower morphology) and the presence of pectinate muscles, trabeculations,

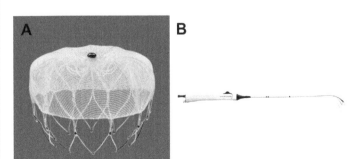

Fig. 1. (*A*) Watchman occlusive device. (*B*) Lariat suture delivery system (*Courtesy of* [*A*] Boston Scientific, Inc., Marlborough, MA; with permission; [*B*] AtriCure, Inc., Mason, OH; with permission.)

lobes, and pouches, which can cause difficulty in endocardial device implantation.[12] LARIAT can accommodate larger appendages (up to 40 mm) but is also limited by LAA morphology. Anatomic exclusions include the following: LAA width greater than 40 mm, superiorly oriented LAA with apex behind PA, multilobed LAA with orientation in different planes exceeding 40 mm, and posteriorly rotated heart.[13–16]

Postprocedural Antithrombotic Therapy

Standard postprocedural antithrombotic therapy exists for the WATCHMAN device as was used in the pivotal clinical trials. Patients are started on warfarin and aspirin for 45 days, at which time a transesophageal echocardiogram (TEE) is performed to evaluate for peridevice leaks and device-related thrombus. If no clots are observed, warfarin is switched to clopidogrel. After 6 months, clopidogrel is discontinued and patients are continued on aspirin.[17] Various other antithrombotic regimens were evaluated in the EWOLUTION (warfarin vs novel oral anticoagulants [NOAC] vs dual antiplatelet therapy [DAPT] versus single antiplatelet therapy [SAPT] versus no therapy), RELEXAO (NOAC vs DAPT vs SAPT vs NOAC plus DAPT vs no therapy), and ASAP (DAPT for 6 months and aspirin indefinitely) studies and continued to demonstrate benefit without difference in outcomes.[18–22] In the EWOLUTION trial, of the 1005 patients included in the study, 60% and 7% received SAPT and DAPT, respectively. Of the remaining patients, 6% were not on anticoagulation, 16% were on vitamin K antagonists (VKA), and 11% were on NOAC (predominantly dabigatran). At 3 months, event rates for device-related thrombus, bleeding rates, and strokes were similar between the groups without statistically significant differences. Interestingly, although NOAC had the lowest numerical event rate, there was no statistical difference demonstrated among any of the studied antithrombotic regimens, including no therapy.[20]

A variety of antithrombotic regimens have been tried for the Amulet device. Tzikas and colleagues[23] used DAPT for up to 1 to 3 months with aspirin 100 mg continued for life. Although there are no manufacturer recommendations regarding the AMPLATZER Amulet, there is a recommendation for ACP, which was followed by Koskinas and colleagues[24] with discontinuation of oral anticoagulants (OAC) following LAAO with DAPT using aspirin 100 mg and clopidogrel 75 mg for at least 5 months and clopidogrel for 1 to 6 months. Korsholm and colleagues[25] attempted to evaluate the efficacy of SAPT with 85% of

patients on aspirin 75 mg monotherapy, 2.8% on clopidogrel 75 mg, and 12.2% on DAPT. The same year, Nielsen-Kudsk and colleagues,[26] attempting to evaluate the efficacy of SAPT in patients with intracranial hemorrhage, had a greater proportion of patients on clopidogrel (31.1%) compared with aspirin (62.1%). The largest Amulet registry to date, by Landmesser and colleagues,[27,28] in which 57.6% of patients are on DAPT, 16.8% are on aspirin, 5.7% are on clopidogrel, 6.6% are on SAPT combined with OAC, 4.6% are on OAC without APT, and 2.1% are without any antithrombotic therapy, reported no significant difference in thromboembolic events.

The LARIAT device has no manufacturer-recommended regimen, and therapy is usually based on clinician discretion. In the initial feasibility study by Bartus and colleagues,[29] patients with contraindications to warfarin remained off warfarin and were on aspirin therapy. In the remaining patients, a standard antithrombotic regimen based on CHADS2 score was used whereby patients with a score of 2 or greater were placed on anticoagulation (warfarin, NOAC), and patients with a score of 1 were placed on aspirin with the decision of anticoagulation based on referring physician's discretion. In a large prospective study conducted by Lakkireddy and colleagues,[30] of the 712 patients enrolled in the study, 79% were off anticoagulation because of prohibitive bleeding risk (67.4%) or high fall risk (11.6%). The remaining 21% were on OAC, either warfarin or DOAC, for at least 6 weeks. Similar to the later WATCHMAN studies, Miller and colleagues[31] in 2014 (comparing aspirin, warfarin, dabigatran, and rivaroxaban) and Price and colleagues[32] in 2016 (comparing aspirin, DAPT, warfarin, rivaroxaban, dabigatran, clopidogrel, aggrenox, and no antithrombotic therapy) used various antithrombotic regimens with the LARIAT system. There were no apparent differences in outcomes among the regimens, but it is important to note that neither study was powered to study differences in outcomes of various regimens.

Stroke Prophylaxis

The PROTECT AF trial was the first prospective RCT that looked at the outcomes of percutaneous LAA closure in comparison to VKA therapy and was published in 2009. It compared the efficacy of the WATCHMAN device to warfarin in 463 patients with a mean follow-up of 18 months. The study demonstrated noninferiority of the WATCHMAN device to warfarin in the primary endpoint, which was a composite of ischemic stroke, cardiovascular or unexplained death, hemorrhagic stroke, and systemic embolism (3% vs 4.9%). The study additionally showed noninferiority in reduction of all strokes (2.3% vs 3.2%), reduction in hemorrhagic stroke (0.2% vs 2.5%), and reduction in all-cause mortality (3.0% vs 4.3%).[18] This study was followed by the PREVAIL study in 2014, which looked at 269 patients undergoing the WATCHMAN procedure and compared its outcomes to 138 patients on VKA therapy over a mean follow-up period of 11.8 months. Although it showed noninferiority in the incidence of late ischemic stroke (after 7 days), the PREVAIL trial failed to demonstrate noninferiority in the composite primary outcome rates.[19] This study brought some of the findings from PROTECT AF into question, prompting further evaluation and limiting probable benefit to the high-risk patient population. Although prophylaxis may have a limited role in lower-stroke-risk patients or those who are not at significant bleeding risk on anticoagulation, patients at high stroke risk (based on CHADS-VaSC score) have a dramatic reduction in risk with the WATCHMAN device. **Table 1** highlights the clinical outcomes data from several large trials and illustrates the efficacy of the WATCHMAN device in this high-risk population.

The AMPLATZER Amulet is a relatively new device in early stages of evaluation but demonstrates promising outcomes. After initial implementation in 2012, small retrospective studies and case reports showed good results prompting involvement in larger trials, typically where outcome data were combined with ACP.[23,25,26,33,34] In 2016, a comparative analysis was released demonstrating a similar short-term complication rate and outcome profile between ACP and Amulet devices.[24] The largest Amulet trial registry to date, which includes 1088 patients, assessed outcomes during a 3-month follow-up. Device implantation rate was 99% with a composite risk of stroke, systemic embolization, and cardiovascular death of 0.6% up to 7 days and 1.4% up to 3 months. A follow-up registry of this same population at 1 year continued to show long-term efficacy, demonstrating a 2.9% stroke risk, a 57% reduction in comparison to predicted stroke risk. Although in early stages of clinical evaluation, the available evidence seems to suggest that the AMPLATZER Amulet offers a similar degree of stroke prophylaxis to WATCHMAN.[27,28] There is an ongoing Amulet-IDE (AMPLATZER Amulet LAA Occluder Trial) clinical trial (NCT02879448) comparing the safety and efficacy of the Amulet device with the WATCHMAN device.

Endocardial occlusion devices appear to have much more robust data supporting claims of stroke prophylaxis compared with epicardial devices. **Table 2** shows notable LARIAT trials and outcomes. The limited population size and mean period of follow-up for patients receiving the LARIAT device make it difficult to draw conclusions. Moreover, the lack of uniformity for LARIAT in postprocedural prophylaxis creates even more difficulty in comparing both devices. In 2015, Pillarisetti and colleagues[35] performed a head-to-head comparison of the LARIAT device with the WATCHMAN device. In their study, even though the patient population with the LARIAT device

Table 1
Large trial trends in WATCHMAN outcomes data

Study	Pilot Study[53]	PROTECT AF[27]	PREVAIL[28]	CAP[47]	EWOLUTION[29]	RELEXAO[30]	ASAP[31]
Patients	75	463	403	460	1019	272	150
Mean follow-up	740 d	18 mo	11.8 mo	0.4 y	30 d	13 mo	14.4 mo
Implant success, %	88	88	95.1	95.0	98.50	96.70	94.70
Pericardial effusion	5	22	1	10	7	0	5
Pleural effusion	0	0	0	0	0	0	0
Stroke	0	6	6	0	3	10	4
Death	2	5	7	0	7	18	9
Site thrombosis	4	0	0	0	0	13	6
Device embolization	2	3	2	0	2	0	2
Major bleeding	1	16	1	3	17	10	0
Average CHADS-VaSC	-	3.5	4	3.9	4.5	4.4	4.4
Expected stroke risk, %	1.9	—	—	—	7.5	—	7.3

Table 2
Trends in LARIAT outcomes data

Study	Bartus et al,[29] 2011	Bartus et al,[42] 2013	Massumi et al,[43] 2013	Price et al,[32] 2014	Miller et al,[31] 2014	Stone et al,[44] 2015	Bartus et al,[45] 2016
Patients	13	89	20	154	41	27	58
Duration	2 mo	1 y	1 y	112 d	3 mo	4 mo	1 y
Implant success, %	92	96	100	94	93	92.6	100
Pericardial effusion	0	1	3	16	18	1	0
Pleural effusion	0	0	0	3	6	1	0
Stroke	0	2	0	2	1	2	0
Procedure-related death	0	1	0	3	0	0	0
Site thrombosis	0	0	0	3	0	1	0
Cardiac perforation	0	0	1	6	4	1	0
Major bleeding	0	0	0	14	2	1	0
Average CHADS/ CHADS-VaSC	—	2.8	4.8	4.1	4.6	5.1	2.75

had both a higher stroke risk and a history of stroke, the LARIAT device provided a similar reduction of transient ischemic attack (TIA)/stroke in comparison to the WATCHMAN device (1.16% vs 1.36%). This study demonstrated that LARIAT had lower incidence of leaks at 1- to 3-month and 9- to 12-month evaluation periods. There was no correlation observed between incidence of leaks and development of thrombus. The investigators then speculate on mechanistic differences in development of leak in LARIAT (central) versus WATCHMAN device (eccentric) that result in different management of leaks. LARIAT leaks are more easily closed using an atrial septal occlusive device (ASO) than leaks with WATCHMAN. There is a need for further RCT comparing devices to understand the differences in outcomes.

Systemic Homeostasis and Neurohormonal Modulation

The LAA produces approximately 30% of the total ANP, but very little is known regarding the LAA neurohormonal impact. In 2015, Maybrook and colleagues[36] presented clinical outcomes of 76 patients who had the LARIAT procedure and found a persistent reduction in systolic blood pressure at 4 to 8 months independent of serum sodium. This study was a precursor for the LAA Homeostasis study, which compared epicardial occlusion and endocardial exclusion with regard to long-term outcomes on neurohormonal modulation. Several key findings can be extracted from the LAA Homeostasis study, as follows:

- An acute reduction in ANP levels postprocedure with epicardial exclusion normalizing at 3 months
- RAAS downregulation persisted through long-term follow-up with epicardial exclusion

Interestingly, these changes were not observed in the endocardial occlusion group, indicating that LAA necrosis after epicardial exclusion plays a crucial role in homeostasis. Postoperative reduction in ANP affects homeostasis via control of volume status and salt balance. After ANP normalizes, persistent RAAS downregulation suggests the LAA may have a role in ANS and RAAS regulation independent of ANP, possibly via the ganglionic plexus (**Fig. 2**). The epicardial approach was demonstrated to have a dramatic reduction in adrenaline, noradrenaline, renin, and aldosterone production that persisted for 3 months postoperatively. In addition, long-term metabolic changes, including increased insulin, free fatty acids, and adiponectin, were observed (**Table 3**). The clinical significance of these metabolic changes and the role of LAA in endocrine modulation is unclear and warrants further investigation. The blood pressure modulation following LAA exclusion has important therapeutic implications for patients with resistant hypertension.[6]

Arrhythmia Management

The success of the Maze procedure, which used LAA excision, in electrical isolation of AF sparked a new interest in the role of LAA in arrhythmia

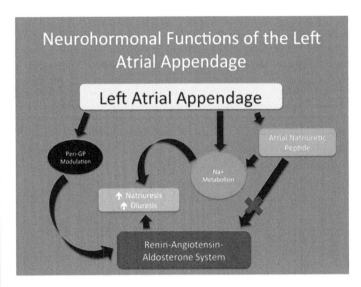

Fig. 2. Impact of LAA on neurohormonal modulation. (*From* Maybrook R, Pillarisetti J, Yarlagadda V, et al. Electrolyte and hemodynamic changes following percutaneous left atrial appendage ligation with the LARIAT device. J Interv Card Electrophysiol. 2015; with permission)

management. Approximately 27% of recurrent AF involves the LAA.[37] LARIAT works similarly to surgical exclusion by inducing LAA necrosis and contributes to electrical isolation of AF. The Left Atrial Appendage Ligation and Ablation for Persistent Atrial Fibrillation Registry involved 138 patients comparing outcomes when ablation for AF was performed alone and in conjunction with LARIAT device placement. At 12 months, patients were 20% more likely to have freedom from atrial tachycardia or AF off antiarrhythmic medications (62% vs 41%). Patients were also half as likely to require repeat ablation (16% vs 33%) with longer median time to AF recurrence (27 weeks vs 19 weeks). The study then evaluated independent predictors of AF and atrial tachycardia recurrence at 12 months using multivariate regression analysis and found that the LARIAT procedure was an

Table 3
Role of left atrial appendage in neurohormonal modulation

| | Impact of LAA Closure Using the Epicardial and Endocardial Devices | | | | | |
| | Postprocedure with Epicardial Device | | | Postprocedure with Endocardial Device | | |
Levels, Compared with Before Procedure:	0 h	24 h	3 mo	0 h	24 h	3 mo
Adrenaline	No change —	↓	↓	—	—	—
Noradrenaline	↓	↓	↓	—	—	—
Aldosterone	—	↓	↓	—	—	—
Renin	—	—	↓	—	—	—
Adioponectin	—	—	↑	—	—	—
Free glycerol levels	—	—	—	—	↓	↓
Insulin	—	↑	↑	—	↑	—
Atrial and brain natriuretic peptides	↓	↑	—	↑	—	—
Systemic blood pressure	↓	↓	↓	↓	—	—

Substantial differences in hemodynamics and neurohormonal impacts. Further studies are required to elucidate the underlying mechanism of these physiologic changes.

The effect of epicardial vs endocardial closure systems on ANP, B-type natriuretic peptide, various components of the renin-angiotensin-aldosterone system, and lipid and glucose metabolism.

Abbreviations: ↑, increased; ↓, decreased.

From Lakkireddy D, Turagam M, Afzal MR, et al. Left Atrial Appendage Closure and Systemic Homeostasis: The LAA HOMEOSTASIS Study. J Am Coll Cardiol. 2018;71(2):135-44; with permission.

independent predictor of recurrence.[38] These small nonrandomized studies laid the groundwork for the much larger randomized aMAZE trial (NCT02513797), a multicenter RCT for the treatment of persistent or longstanding persistent AF. This trial will determine the safety and efficacy of using ablation plus adjunctive percutaneous endoepicardial exclusion. There are currently 53 active sites and a goal of 600 patients with an estimated completion date of December 2019/January 2020. Preliminary data from this trial have showed promising results. There are no current data supporting electrical isolation of AF with the use of endocardial occlusion devices.

Device-Related Complications

Leaks

Although mention of leaks and peridevice flow in original trials appears to be less commonly found, a post hoc analysis of the PROTECT-AF data found a 32% incidence of peridevice flow.[39] A similar incidence of leaks was noted in follow-up of patients with ACP. A comparison study of the ACP with the Amulet device over a 3-month follow-up period found a significant reduction in incidence of leaks (48% vs 8%).[40] In 2015, Saw and colleagues[41] used cardiac computed tomography angiography (CCTA) to assess for the presence of residual leaks comparing the ACP, the AMPLATZER Amulet, and the WATCHMAN device at 3-month follow-up. They found a much higher incidence of leaks than previously reported (70.6% vs 66.7% vs 55.6%, respectively) without any statistically significant difference between the 3 devices. CCTA was likely responsible for increased incidence of leaks in this study because this method is more sensitive than TEE. There were 3 major

hypotheses for the development of leaks with endocardial occlusion based on this analysis: absence of perpendicularity between landing zone and device resulting in mismatch, gap related to lack of device expansion against landing zone wall, and absence of device seal with consequent incomplete endothelialization.

Incidence of leaks in the LARIAT device can also vary, acute leaks noted in 0% to 8%, early leaks (<6 months) noted in 5% to 24%, and late leaks (6–12 months) noted in 2% to 20%.[31,32,42–45] In a head-to-head comparison of WATCHMAN and LARIAT at a 9- to 12-month follow-up, WATCHMAN was found to have a higher leak incidence (21% vs 13%) and leak size (3.10 mm vs 2.15 mm). The mechanisms of leak development in WATCHMAN and LARIAT are fundamentally different and have management implications. WATCHMAN develops leaks via the Edge effect, based on positional changes and local tissue remodeling consequently resulting in an eccentric leak. LARIAT develops leaks via the gunnysack effect: diverticula in the excluded appendage, which contributes toward loosening of the closure resulting in a consequent concentric leak (**Fig. 3**). Concentric leaks are more easily closed with ASO, although there are case reports describing the use of the ASO device to close eccentric leaks. Typically, eccentric leaks are more difficult to close and require the use of anticoagulation, likely negating the benefit of using LAA closure devices.[35] Currently, no robust evidence to support the relationship of peridevice flow and development of thromboembolism in percutaneous devices is available.[39] Much of the available literature regarding leak size and thrombogenicity is from publications on surgical exclusion. Typically, leaks larger than 5 mm are considered to be high risk.

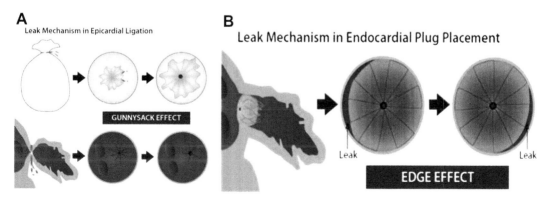

Fig. 3. (A) Mechanism of gunnysack effect. (B) Mechanism of edge effect. (From Pillarisetti J, Reddy YM, Gunda S, et al. Endocardial (Watchman) vs epicardial (Lariat) left atrial appendage exclusion devices: Understanding the differences in the location and type of leaks and their clinical implications. Heart Rhythm. 2015; with permission.)

Table 4
Upcoming clinical trials and expected completion dates

Device	Upcoming Recruiting, Enrolling, Active Trials (Expected Completion)
Endocardial devices	
AMPLATZER Cardiac Plug	• Postapproval Study (PAS) (10/2023) • PAS China (12/2023)
AMPLATZER Amulet	• Prevention of Stroke by Left Atrial Appendage Closure in Atrial Fibrillation Patients After Intracerebral Hemorrhage (5/2030) • Optimal Antiplatelet Treatment to Achieve Stroke Avoidance and Fall in Bleeding Events Following Left Atrial Appendage Closure (SAFE-LAAC). Comparative Health Effectiveness Randomized Trial–PILOT Study (1/2022) • Postapproval Study of Percutaneous Left Atrial Appendage Closure: FLAAC-2 (Comparing WATCHMAN, ACP, and Amulet) (6/2021) • AMPLATZER Amulet Left Atrial Appendage Occluder Randomized Controlled Trial (Amulet IDE) (12/2023)
WAveCrest	• WAveCrest vs WATCHMAN TranssEptal LAA Closure to REduce AF-Mediated STroke 2 (WAVECREST2) (12/2025)
LAmbre	• Left Atrial Appendage Occlusion in Patients with Nonvalvular Atrial Fibrillation From Shanghai (LAAO-SH; Comparing LAmbre, Lefort, Leftear, and WATCHMAN) (6/2020) • Lifetech LAmbre Left Atrial Appendage (LAA) Closure System Post-market Clinical Follow-up (8/2022)
WATCHMAN	• WATCH-TAVR, WATCHMAN for Patients With Atrial Fibrillation Undergoing Transcatheter Aortic Valve Replacement (12/2020) • China REgistry of WATCHMAN (9/2020) • WATCHMAN for Second Prevention of Stroke (WASPS) (11/2020) • Latin America Registry on WATCHMAN Outcomes in Real Life (12/2018) • Left Atrial Appendage Occlusion With WATCHMAN Device in Patients with Nonvalvular Atrial Fibrillation and End-stage Chronic Kidney Disease on Hemodialysis (3/2021) • WAveCrest vs WATCHMAN TranssEptal LAA Closure to REduce AF-Mediated STroke 2 (WAVECREST2) (12/2025) • Efficacy of Short Term Dabigatran Etexilate Followed by Aspirin Monotherapy After LAA (Left Atrial Appendage) Device Closure (the DEA-LAA Study) (8/2020) • A Pilot Study of Edoxaban in Patients with Nonvalvular Atrial Fibrillation and Left Atrial Appendage Closure (12/2019) • Left Atrial Appendage Occlusion vs Novel Oral Anticoagulation for Stroke Prevention in Atrial Fibrillation (10/2030) • Left Atrial Appendage Occlusion in Patients with Nonvalvular Atrial Fibrillation From Shanghai (6/2020) • Postapproval Study of Percutaneous Left Atrial Appendage Closure (FLAAC-2) (6/2021) • Left Atrial Appendage Closure vs Novel Anticoagulation Agents in Atrial Fibrillation (5/2020) • Assessment of the WATCHMAN Device in Patients Unsuitable for Oral Anticoagulation (12/2023)
WATCHMAN FLX	• Comparison of Anticoagulation With Left Atrial Appendage Closure After AF Ablation (9/2021) • WATCHMAN FLX Left Atrial Appendage Closure Device Postapproval Study (Europe Only) (7/2021)
Lefort	• Left Atrial Appendage Occlusion in Patients with Nonvalvular Atrial Fibrillation From Shanghai (LAAO-SH; Comparing LAmbre, Lefort, Leftear, and WATCHMAN) (6/2020)
Leftear	• Left Atrial Appendage Occlusion in Patients with Nonvalvular Atrial Fibrillation From Shanghai (LAAO-SH; Comparing LAmbre, Lefort, Leftear, and WATCHMAN) (6/2020)

(continued on next page)

Table 4
(continued)

Device	Upcoming Recruiting, Enrolling, Active Trials (Expected Completion)
Epicardial devices	
LARIAT	• aMAZE Study: LAA Ligation Adjunctive to PVI for Persistent or Longstanding Persistent Atrial Fibrillation (12/2019)
Atriclip	• Stand-alone Totally Thoracoscopic Left Atrial Appendage Occlusion Using AtriClip Device in Nonvalvular Atrial Fibrillation (1/2025) • AtriCure CryoICE Lesions for Persistent and Long-standing Persistent Atrial Fibrillation Treatment (1/2023) • Pivotal Study of a Dual Epicardial & Endocardial Procedure (DEEP) Approach (12/2025) • Combined Endoscopic Epicardial and Percutaneous Endocardial Ablation vs Repeated Catheter Ablation in Persistent and Long-standing Persistent Atrial Fibrillation (11/2020)

Device/site thrombus

Site thrombosis was a major reason incomplete closure resulted in worse outcomes in surgical exclusion. In evaluation of major trial data for WATCHMAN and LARIAT, it appears as though risk of site thrombus formation is uncommon. A recent systematic review using multiple smaller trials found WATCHMAN, ACP, and Amulet to have a range of device-related thrombosis (DRT) rate of 0% to 8.2% for studies involving 100 or more patients. Although mean pooled incidence of DRT was 3.9%, subdivision showed 3.4% for WATCHMAN, 4.6% for ACP/Amulet, 4.8% for ACP, and 2% for Amulet. Incidence of DRT 6 weeks postoperatively (which was also the mean time to diagnosis) was similar between WATCHMAN and ACP/Amulet (2% vs 2.6%, $P = .6$). Collectively, 0.28% of patients with implant and DRT had resultant stroke or TIA; however, most cases (94%) were asymptomatic.[46] The RELEXAO Registry provided a unique insight on WATCHMAN device outcomes in high-risk patient populations. In the RELEXAO Registry, site thrombosis was noted in 7.2% of the patients, which was significantly higher than the previously reported 3.9%. They highlighted a strong association of device thrombosis with stroke and TIA.[21]

Cardiac puncture and pericardial effusion

A known complication of the WATCHMAN device is pericardial effusions. Overall incidence of pericardial effusions is between 0% and 6.7% based on major trial data, although individual study rates have a high degree of variability. It should be noted, however, that early trials had high rates of effusion, and this decreased over time. As seen in the CAP Registry, this was a likely result of improved operator experience.[47] A similar rate of pericardial effusions is observed in smaller trial Amulet data ranging from 0% to 4%.[28,40,48,49] Registry data from Landmesser and colleagues[28] show an incidence of 1.65%. The epicardial access required for the LARIAT device on the other hand predisposes patients to the complications of cardiac puncture and pericardial effusion. Smaller sampling size and high variability of perioperative management strategy (ie, micropuncture needle, use of second-generation LARIAT device, colchicine prophylaxis) are likely responsible for variability of observed rates of pericardial effusion (0%–44%). Even after excluding the major outlier (Miller and colleagues), the incidence remains high at 0% to 15%. Prophylaxis appears to be a good strategy for prevention and reduction in severity of pericardial effusion. Although variable, some successful prevention strategies include the use of micropuncture needle, nonsteroidal anti-inflammatory drugs, intrapericardial steroids, periprocedural colchicine, and pericardial drain in situ.[30,50]

Device embolization

Intracardiac device placement raises a concern for the risk of embolization. Typically, to avoid this complication, devices are oversized. The WATCHMAN device additionally has barbs to ensure proper fitting after implantation. Post hoc analysis of WATCHMAN data from PROTECT AF and EWOLUTION trials reveals incidence of device

Table 5
LARIAT versus WATCHMAN procedural differences

Device	LARIAT[29,31,42]	WATCHMAN[47,54]
Procedural time (min)	45–127	50–82
Fluoroscopy time (min)	13.6–16.2	25–47

Table 6
LARIAT and WATCHMAN statistically significant outcome differences from MAUDE database

	Pre-FDA WATCHMAN, %	Post-FDA WATCHMAN, %	WATCHMAN, %	LARIAT, %
Pericardiocentesis	0.2	1.39	0.98	0.47
Device embolization	0.05	0.68	—	—
Cardiac surgery	0.05	0.94	—	—
Device malfunction	0.1	2.49	1.66	0.18

Adapted from Jazayeri MA, Vuddanda V, Turagam MK, et al. Safety profiles of percutaneous left atrial appendage closure devices: An analysis of the Food and Drug Administration Manufacturer and User Facility Device Experience (MAUDE) database from 2009 to 2016. J Cardiovasc Electrophysiol. 2018; with permission.

embolization to be 0.6% to 2.7%.[39,51] For the WATCHMAN and Amulet devices, the greatest embolization incidence occurred within 24 hours, whereas the WATCHMAN also had a relatively high rate of embolization after 1 week. This study characterized embolization as complicated (requiring surgery, requiring vascular repair, or resulting in valvular damage, end organ damage, or death) and noncomplicated. Noncomplicated embolizations generally occurred in the LA. Embolizations that occurred further along the postoperative course generally correlated with the need for surgery. On evaluation of common reasons for embolization, top reasons appeared to be LAA size-device mismatch, anatomic issues (flat landing zone, chicken-wing anatomy, multiple lobes, scanty trabeculations, prominent pectinate muscles, and funnel entrance), operator dependence, conversion to sinus rhythm after device deployment, and concomitant radiofrequency ablation resulting in inflammatory changes at the ridge. No obvious reason for embolization was seen in 64% of cases. Although oversizing can help to reduce the incidence of postoperative device embolization, this approach has limited utility. Overcompression can push the device out of position (watermelon seed effect). In addition, up to one-third of WATCHMAN devices appear to lose compression over time.[52,53]

SUMMARY

Although the endocardial approach allows us to directly address thromboembolic risk, the necrosis that occurs as a consequence of epicardial ligation appears to address the arrhythmia itself and conditions responsible for the propagation and continuation of the disease. As the understanding of the mechanistic and technical difference between both approaches continues to expand, physicians will be better equipped to tailor management toward patient-specific needs (**Tables 4–6**).

DISCLOSURE

The authors have no relationship with a commercial company that has a direct financial interest in the subject matter or materials discussed in this article.

REFERENCES

1. Blackshear JL, Odell JA. Appendage obliteration to reduce stroke in cardiac surgical patients with atrial fibrillation. Ann Thorac Surg 1996;61(2):755–9.
2. Goldman ME, Pearce LA, Hart RG, et al. Pathophysiologic correlates of thromboembolism in nonvalvular atrial fibrillation: I. Reduced flow velocity in the left atrial appendage (The Stroke Prevention in Atrial Fibrillation [SPAF-III] study). J Am Soc Echocardiogr 1999;12:1080–7.
3. Akoum N, Fernandez G, Wilson B, et al. Association of atrial fibrosis quantified using LGE-MRI with atrial appendage thrombus and spontaneous contrast on transesophageal echocardiography in patients with atrial fibrillation. J Cardiovasc Electrophysiol 2013; 24:1104–9.
4. Iwasaki YK, Nishida K, Kato T, et al. Atrial fibrillation pathophysiology: implications for management. Circulation 2011. https://doi.org/10.1161/CIRCULATIONAHA.111.019893.
5. Naksuk N, Padmanabhan D, Yogeswaran V, et al. Left atrial appendage: embryology, anatomy, physiology, arrhythmia and therapeutic intervention. JACC Clin Electrophysiol 2016. https://doi.org/10.1016/j.jacep.2016.06.006.
6. Lakkireddy D, Turagam M, Afzal MR, et al. Left atrial appendage closure and systemic homeostasis: the LAA HOMEOSTASIS study. J Am Coll Cardiol 2018. https://doi.org/10.1016/j.jacc.2017.10.092.
7. Tabata T, Oki T, Yamada H, et al. Role of left atrial appendage in left atrial reservoir function as evaluated by left atrial appendage clamping during cardiac surgery. Am J Cardiol 1998;81:327–32.
8. Leinonen JV, Emanuelov AK, Platt Y, et al. Left atrial appendages from adult hearts contain a reservoir of diverse cardiac progenitor cells. PLoS One 2013;8: e59228.

9. Mahilmaran A, Nayar PG, Sudarsana G, et al. Relationship of left atrial appendage function to left ventricular function. Indian Heart J 2004;56:293–8.

10. Kreidieh B, Rojas F, Schurmann P, et al. Left atrial appendage remodeling after Lariat left atrial appendage ligation. Circ Arrhythm Electrophysiol 2015. https://doi.org/10.1161/CIRCEP.115.003188.

11. Kawamura M, Scheinman MM, Lee RJ, et al. Left atrial appendage ligation in patients with atrial fibrillation leads to a decrease in atrial dispersion. J Am Heart Assoc 2015;4 [pii:e001581].

12. Turagam MK, Velagapudi P, Kar S, et al. Cardiovascular therapies targeting left atrial appendage. J Am Coll Cardiol 2018. https://doi.org/10.1016/j.jacc.2018.05.048.

13. Srivastava MC, See VY, Dawood MY, et al. A review of the LARIAT device: insights from the cumulative clinical experience. Springerplus 2015. https://doi.org/10.1186/s40064-015-1289-8.

14. Asmarats L, Rodés-Cabau J. Percutaneous left atrial appendage closure: current devices and clinical outcomes. Circ Cardiovasc Interv 2017. https://doi.org/10.1161/CIRCINTERVENTIONS.117.005359.

15. Saw J, Lempereur M. Percutaneous left atrial appendage closure procedural techniques and outcomes. JACC Cardiovasc Interv 2014. https://doi.org/10.1016/j.jcin.2014.05.026.

16. Litwinowicz R, Bartus M, Burysz M, et al. Long term outcomes after left atrial appendage closure with the LARIAT device—stroke risk reduction over five years follow-up. PLoS One 2018. https://doi.org/10.1371/journal.pone.0208710.

17. "WATCHMAN™ left atrial appendage closure device." Patient information guide, Boston Scientific. Available at: www.accessdata.fda.gov/cdrh_docs/pdf13/P130013c.pdf. Accessed August 1, 2019.

18. Holmes DR, Reddy VY, Turi ZG, et al. Percutaneous closure of the left atrial appendage versus warfarin therapy for prevention of stroke in patients with atrial fibrillation: a randomised non-inferiority trial. Lancet 2009. https://doi.org/10.1016/S0140-6736(09)61343-X.

19. Holmes DR, Kar S, Price MJ, et al. Prospective randomized evaluation of the Watchman left Atrial appendage closure device in patients with atrial fibrillation versus long-term Warfarin therapy: the PREVAIL trial. J Am Coll Cardiol 2014;64(1):1–12.

20. Boersma LV, Ince H, Kische S, et al. Efficacy and safety of left atrial appendage closure with WATCHMAN in patients with or without contraindication to oral anticoagulation: 1-year follow-up outcome data of the EWOLUTION trial. Hear Rhythm 2017. https://doi.org/10.1016/j.hrthm.2017.05.038.

21. Fauchier L, Cinaud A, Brigadeau F, et al. Device-related thrombosis after percutaneous left atrial appendage occlusion for atrial fibrillation. J Am Coll Cardiol 2018. https://doi.org/10.1016/j.jacc.2018.01.076.

22. Reddy VY, Möbius-Winkler S, Miller MA, et al. Left atrial appendage closure with the Watchman device in patients with a contraindication for oral anticoagulation: the ASAP study (ASA plavix feasibility study with Watchman left atrial appendage closure technology). J Am Coll Cardiol 2013. https://doi.org/10.1016/j.jacc.2013.03.035.

23. Tzikas A, Karagounis L, Bouktsi M, et al. Left atrial appendage occlusion with the Amplatzer Amulet™ for stroke prevention in atrial fibrillation: the first case in Greece. Hellenic J Cardiol 2013;54(5):408–12.

24. Koskinas KC, Shakir S, Fankhauser M, et al. Predictors of early (1-week) outcomes following left atrial appendage closure with Amplatzer devices. JACC Cardiovasc Interv 2016. https://doi.org/10.1016/j.jcin.2016.04.019.

25. Korsholm K, Nielsen KM, Jensen JM, et al. Transcatheter left atrial appendage occlusion in patients with atrial fibrillation and a high bleeding risk using aspirin alone for post-implant antithrombotic therapy. EuroIntervention 2017. https://doi.org/10.4244/EIJ-D-16-00726.

26. Nielsen-Kudsk JE, Johnsen SP, Wester P, et al. Left atrial appendage occlusion versus standard medical care in patients with atrial fibrillation and intracerebral haemorrhage: a propensity score-matched follow-up study. EuroIntervention 2017. https://doi.org/10.4244/EIJ-D-17-00201.

27. Landmesser U, Schmidt B, Nielsen-Kudsk JE, et al. Left atrial appendage occlusion with the AMPLATZER Amulet device: periprocedural and early clinical/echocardiographic data from a global prospective observational study. EuroIntervention 2017. https://doi.org/10.4244/EIJ-D-17-00493.

28. Landmesser U, Tondo C, Camm J, et al. Left atrial appendage occlusion with the AMPLATZER Amulet device: one-year follow-up from the prospective global Amulet observational registry. EuroIntervention 2018. https://doi.org/10.4244/EIJ-D-18-00344.

29. Bartus K, Bednarek J, Myc J, et al. Feasibility of closed-chest ligation of the left atrial appendage in humans. Hear Rhythm 2011. https://doi.org/10.1016/j.hrthm.2010.10.040.

30. Lakkireddy D, Afzal MR, Lee RJ, et al. Short and long-term outcomes of percutaneous left atrial appendage suture ligation: results from a US multicenter evaluation. Hear Rhythm 2016. https://doi.org/10.1016/j.hrthm.2016.01.022.

31. Miller MA, Gangireddy SR, Doshi SK, et al. Multicenter study on acute and long-term safety and efficacy of percutaneous left atrial appendage closure using an epicardial suture snaring device. Hear Rhythm 2014. https://doi.org/10.1016/j.hrthm.2014.07.032.

32. Price MJ, Gibson DN, Yakubov SJ, et al. Early safety and efficacy of percutaneous left atrial appendage suture ligation: results from the U.S. Transcatheter LAA ligation consortium. J Am Coll Cardiol 2014. https://doi.org/10.1016/j.jacc.2014.03.057.

33. Freixa X, Chan JLK, Tzikas A, et al. The Amplatzer Cardiac Plug 2 for left atrial appendage occlusion: novel features and first-in-man experience. EuroIntervention 2013. https://doi.org/10.4244/EIJV8I9A167.

34. Lam SCC, Bertog S, Gafoor S, et al. Left atrial appendage closure using the Amulet device: an initial experience with the second generation Amplatzer cardiac plug. Catheter Cardiovasc Interv 2015. https://doi.org/10.1002/ccd.25644.

35. Pillarisetti J, Reddy YM, Gunda S, et al. Endocardial (Watchman) vs epicardial (Lariat) left atrial appendage exclusion devices: understanding the differences in the location and type of leaks and their clinical implications. Hear Rhythm 2015. https://doi.org/10.1016/j.hrthm.2015.03.020.

36. Maybrook R, Pillarisetti J, Yarlagadda V, et al. Electrolyte and hemodynamic changes following percutaneous left atrial appendage ligation with the LARIAT device. J Interv Card Electrophysiol 2015. https://doi.org/10.1007/s10840-015-0012-6.

37. Di Biase L, Burkhardt JD, Mohanty P, et al. Left atrial appendage: an underrecognized trigger site of atrial fibrillation. Circulation 2010. https://doi.org/10.1161/CIRCULATIONAHA.109.928903.

38. Lakkireddy D, Sridhar Mahankali A, Kanmanthareddy A, et al. Left atrial appendage ligation and ablation for persistent atrial fibrillation: the LAALA-AF registry. JACC Clin Electrophysiol 2015. https://doi.org/10.1016/j.jacep.2015.04.006.

39. Viles-Gonzalez JF, Kar S, Douglas P, et al. The clinical impact of incomplete left atrial appendage closure with the Watchman device in patients with atrial fibrillation: a PROTECT AF (Percutaneous Closure of the Left Atrial Appendage Versus Warfarin Therapy for Prevention of Stroke in Patients with Atrial Fibrillation) substudy. J Am Coll Cardiol 2012. https://doi.org/10.1016/j.jacc.2011.11.028.

40. Abualsaud A, Freixa X, Tzikas A, et al. Side-by-side comparison of LAA occlusion performance with the Amplatzer cardiac plug and Amplatzer Amulet. J Invasive Cardiol 2016;28(1):34–8.

41. Saw J, Fahmy P, DeJong P, et al. Cardiac CT angiography for device surveillance after endovascular left atrial appendage closure. Eur Heart J Cardiovasc Imaging 2015. https://doi.org/10.1093/ehjci/jev067.

42. Bartus K, Han FT, Bednarek J, et al. Percutaneous left atrial appendage suture ligation using the Lariat device in patients with atrial fibrillation: initial clinical experience. J Am Coll Cardiol 2013. https://doi.org/10.1016/j.jacc.2012.06.046.

43. Massumi A, Chelu MG, Nazeri A, et al. Initial experience with a novel percutaneous left atrial appendage exclusion device in patients with atrial fibrillation, increased stroke risk, and contraindications to anticoagulation. Am J Cardiol 2013. https://doi.org/10.1016/j.amjcard.2012.11.061.

44. Stone D, Byrne T, Pershad A. Early results with the LARIAT device for left atrial appendage exclusion in patients with atrial fibrillation at high risk for stroke and anticoagulation. Catheter Cardiovasc Interv 2015. https://doi.org/10.1002/ccd.25065.

45. Bartus K, Gafoor S, Tschopp D, et al. Left atrial appendage ligation with the next generation LARIAT+ suture delivery device: early clinical experience. Int J Cardiol 2016. https://doi.org/10.1016/j.ijcard.2016.04.005.

46. Lempereur M, Aminian A, Freixa X, et al. Device-associated thrombus formation after left atrial appendage occlusion: a systematic review of events reported with the Watchman, the Amplatzer Cardiac Plug and the Amulet. Catheter Cardiovasc Interv 2017;90(5):E111–21.

47. Phillips KP, Walker DT, Humphries JA. Combined catheter ablation for atrial fibrillation and Watchman left atrial appendage occlusion procedures: five-year experience. J Arrhythm 2016. https://doi.org/10.1016/j.joa.2015.11.001.

48. Kleinecke C, Park JW, Gödde M, et al. Twelve-month follow-up of left atrial appendage occlusion with Amplatzer Amulet. Cardiol J 2017. https://doi.org/10.5603/CJ.a2017.0017.

49. Freixa X, Abualsaud A, Chan J, et al. Left atrial appendage occlusion: initial experience with the Amplatzer™ Amulet™. Int J Cardiol 2014. https://doi.org/10.1016/j.ijcard.2014.03.154.

50. Dar, Turagam, Yarlagadda, et al. "Managing Pericardium in Electrophysiology Procedures." American College of Cardiology, Latest in Cardiology: Expert Opinion, 27 Oct. 2017. Available at: www.acc.org/latest-in-cardiology/articles/2017/10/27/10/20/managing-pericardium-in-electrophysiology-procedures. Accessed August 14, 2019.

51. Boersma LVA, Schmidt B, Betts TR, et al. Implant success and safety of left atrial appendage closure with the WATCHMAN device: peri-procedural outcomes from the EWOLUTION registry. Eur Heart J 2016. https://doi.org/10.1093/eurheartj/ehv730.

52. Dar T, Yarlagadda B, Tzikas A, et al. Left atrial appendage occlusion device embolization (LAAODE): understanding the timing, mechanism, and outcomes. J Am Coll Cardiol 2018. https://doi.org/10.1016/s0735-1097(18)30943-4.

53. Sick PB, Schuler G, Hauptmann KE, et al. Initial worldwide experience with the WATCHMAN left atrial appendage system for stroke prevention in atrial fibrillation. J Am Coll Cardiol 2007. https://doi.org/10.1016/j.jacc.2007.02.035.

54. Reddy VY, Holmes D, Doshi SK, et al. Safety of percutaneous left atrial appendage closure: results from the watchman left atrial appendage system for embolic protection in patients with AF (PROTECT AF) clinical trial and the continued access registry. Circulation 2011. https://doi.org/10.1161/CIRCULATIONAHA.110.976449.

Current State of Surgical Left Atrial Appendage Exclusion: How and When

James R. Edgerton, MD, FHRS

KEYWORDS

• Atrial fibrillation • Left atrial appendage • Stroke • Cardiac surgery • Left atrial appendage exclusion

KEY POINTS

• Left atrial appendage exclusion is efficacious for stroke prophylaxis in patients with atrial fibrillation.
• Surgical excision provides reliable left atrial appendage exclusion, whereas surgical occlusion does not. Specifically, 2-layer internally suture ligation has a high failure rate.
• Left atrial appendage exclusion concomitant to another cardiac surgical procedure is indicated in patients with atrial fibrillation but not in patients without baseline atrial fibrillation.
• Studies currently underway will further define the role of concomitant surgical left atrial appendage exclusion, especially for the population without baseline atrial fibrillation but at high risk of developing postoperative atrial fibrillation.

INTRODUCTION

Stroke is often a disabling condition. Between 15% and 20% of strokes are related to atrial fibrillation (AF) and the risk of stroke is 5 times greater in patients with AF compared with those without AF.[1] These strokes related to AF tend to be the most disabling, with 31% being fatal and another 39% resulting in moderate or severe disability.[2,3] Although treatment with an oral anticoagulant can be effective, at any given time, only 55% of people treated with warfarin are in the therapeutic range.[4] In addition, compliance rates in patients treated with a novel oral anticoagulant at 1.3 years are approximately 60% even with apixaban. It is further known that, in nonvalvular AF, the left atrial appendage (LAA) is the most common site of thrombus formation and these thrombi are causal in 57% of non–rheumatic-related and 91% of rheumatic AF–related strokes.[5,6] All this caused Johnson and colleagues[7] to label the LAA as "…our most lethal human attachment!" Therefore, in an effort to reduce AF-related stroke, the LAA has been targeted for occlusion by many clincians.[8,9] Removal of the LAA for stroke prophylaxis was first reported in 1948,[10] but perhaps the first concerted effort in a series to eliminate the LAA from circulation was by Cox and colleagues,[11] concomitant with a Maze procedure. In an 8.5-year follow-up of 164 patients, 2 had transient ischemic attacks and there were no ischemic strokes. Specific to the mitral valve, in 2003 García-Fernández and colleagues[12] performed a retrospective study of 205 patients with previous mitral valve replacement and echocardiography at 69.4 ± 67 months. The main outcome measure was an embolic event, more than 48 hours after surgery. They concluded that LAA ligation during mitral valve replacement is consistent with a 6.7-fold reduction in the risk of late embolism. If a complete LAA ligation is achieved and confirmed with transesophageal echocardiogram (TEE), a further reduction in embolism risk is observed (11.9-fold reduction).

More recently, in large prospective randomized trials, elimination of the LAA has been shown conclusively to be effective prophylaxis against stroke in patients with AF.[9,13,14] Mounting evidence such as these and other publications[15]

Department of Epidemiology, Baylor Scott and White Health, PO Box 190667, Dallas, TX 75219, USA
E-mail address: JamesEdgertonMD@gmail.com

Card Electrophysiol Clin 12 (2020) 109–115
https://doi.org/10.1016/j.ccep.2019.10.001
1877-9182/20/© 2019 Elsevier Inc. All rights reserved.

has led to several societal recommendations for surgical management of the LAA in patients with AF undergoing cardiac surgery for another cause. Both the 2016 European Society of Cardiology[16] and the 2014 American Heart Association/American College of Cardiology[17] guidelines give class IIb recommendations, and the more recent 2017 Society of Thoracic Surgeons (STS) guideline[18] gives a class IIa recommendation for closure.

Surgeons have been routinely eliminating the LAA during mitral valve surgery since the work of Madden[10] in 1948, mentioned earlier. Surgical management of the LAA has been performed by epicardial suture ligation (oversew, purse string), endocardial suture ligation, stapler exclusion, stapler excision (±reinforcement), snares/suture loops, and epicardial exclusion clips. The varied effectiveness of these techniques in eliminating the LAA from the systemic circulation accounts for the checkered past of surgical management. Thus, when studying the efficacy of surgical LAA elimination for stroke prophylaxis, it is first necessary to know which surgical technique was used and its relative efficacy in eliminating the appendage from the circulation.

METHODS OF SURGICAL CLOSURE AND SUCCESS RATE
Lack of Efficacy of Suture and Staple Closure

Multiple series have shown that most of the methods historically used to close the LAA result in incomplete closure. Chief among these (but not alone) is endocardial suture closure without amputation. This method was initially done with a single encircling purse string suture but, as the high failure rate of this became generally known, most surgeons changed to single-layer or double-layer running suture closure thinking this more efficacious. However, in 2000 Katz and colleagues[19] showed that this technique has a 36% failure rate. They reviewed 50 patients who had endocardial LAA closure concomitant to a mitral operation and who were studied by early and/or late echocardiogram. Thirty-six percent had incomplete exclusion. Among these, 50% had thrombus or spontaneous echo contrast (SEC) and 22% sustained thromboembolism. In contrast, Natale and colleagues assessed the risk of oral anticoagulation (OAC) in 191 patients with AF with LAA clip closure. Patients underwent TEE at 1 and 6 months and follow-up was 16.7 ± 8.5 months. They found that 87.3% had some proximal smooth-walled neck below the clip but there was no LAA thrombus. One patient (0.5%) who also had amyloid vasculitis sustained a stroke and 3 patients (1.57%) had a transient

ischemic attack (TIA), but each of these had a left atrial diameter greater than 6 cm and SEC.[20] In the Left Atrial Appendage Occlusion Study (LAAOS), 52 patients were randomized to staple or suture closure and assessed by TEE. Failure was defined as a residual stump larger than 1 cm or residual flow into the LAA. There was only 45% successful occlusion by suture and 72% successful closure by stapler.[21]

Excision Versus Exclusion

Careful examination of the literature reveals efficacy differences between exclusion and excision of the LAA, with the latter being more effective. In a well-known 2008 study, Kanderian and colleagues[22] reported TEE assessment of LAA closure by 3 different techniques. Success followed the usual definition of no residual flow into the LAA and no stump larger than 1 cm. Excision had a markedly better success rate than exclusion (**Table 1**) by either suture techniques or a noncutting stapler.[22] None of the excised appendages had thrombus at the base or in the stump, whereas this was common in the excluded appendages.

A 2015 study examined 75 patients who underwent 2-layer oversewn LAA closure concomitant to a mitral valve and ablation procedure. On computed tomography (CT) scan performed at 3 months or later, 35% had incomplete closure.[23]

Note that surgical staplers can be subdivided into those that staple closed the base and those that staple closed the base and amputate the distal remnant. Stapling without amputation uniformly fails, as is shown in the study referenced earlier, as well as others.[24]

Lee and colleagues[25] reported late neurologic events in 710 patients who underwent LAA excision versus those who underwent alternative closure techniques between 2004 and 2011. The

Table 1 Success of left atrial appendage closure by 3 techniques. Exclusion techniques recanalize over time	
Surgical Technique	**Successful Management (%)**
Excision	73
Exclusion (suture)	23
Exclusion (non cutting stapler)	0

Data from Kanderian AS, Gillinov, AM, Patterson GB, et al. Success of surgical left atrial appendage closure: assessment by transesophageal echo. JACC 2008;52(11):924-29.

rate of late neurologic event was 1.13% in those who underwent alternative elimination versus 0.2% in patients who underwent LAA excision ($P = .001$).[25]

In reviewing the literature, the pattern emerges that appendages that are excluded by any suture technique or by noncutting stapling recanalize over time as the sutures and the staples erode through the endothelialized surfaces. An analogous situation exists in gastrointestinal surgery, in which closures across mucosally lined viscera recanalize over time. The essential element seems to be excision,[26] which leaves 2 raw edges to scar together. The exception to this observation of higher success of excision versus exclusion is external clip closure, because the closure pressure of the clip results in a line of necrosis between the closure elements, and the distal LAA is commonly observed to immediately become cyanotic on clip application. The closure members of this clip are titanium tubes inside carbothane pressure pads and covered with polyester. Confirmatory of this closure pressure is the fact that application of the AtriClip (AtriCure, West Chester, OH) results in immediate total electrical isolation of the LAA.[27] In a pivotal trial, 61 patients with an AtriClip were studied with TEE or CT at 3 months. Sixty of 61 patients (98.4%) has successful occlusion. No patient had residual flow but 1 had a residual stump larger than 1 cm accounting for the single failure caused by improper placement.[28] In a subsequent study, 40 patients were followed with CT at baseline and at 3, 12, 24, and 36 months. Average follow-up was 3.5 ± 0.5 years. At 36 months, all clips were stable with no displacement, no intracardiac thrombi, no LAA perfused, no residual neck larger than 1 cm, no strokes, and no TIAs or neurologic events.[29]

Thus, the common denominator for successful surgical exclusion of the LAA is excision. The single exception to this is application of an external clip device, which mimics excision because its closing pressure induces necrosis of the distal appendage.

STAND-ALONE SURGICAL CLOSURE

Surgeons have traditionally called operations done solely for AF or to close the LAA lone-AF procedures. However, in the electrophysiology world, lone AF refers to AF that exists in the absence of any structural heart disease. Accordingly, the 2017 Consensus Statement[30] recommended that surgeons and surgical literature adopt the term stand-alone to refer to AF and LAA procedures that are not concomitant with another cardiac operation.

Stand-alone surgery for LAA exclusion has historically found only very limited application because of the associated morbidity related to access trauma. However, with the advent of enabling technology, stand-alone LAA closure can be accomplished thoracoscopically using 3 small ports in the left chest.[31] This procedure can be accomplished in 30 minutes without the use of intraoperative or postoperative anticoagulation. Thus, it may be the procedure of choice for frail patients who have a contraindication to anticoagulation.

The LAA has numerous anatomic presentations and can be categorized into one of 4 groups based on its anatomy on CT scan (cactus, cauliflower, chicken wing, and windsock), and cauliflower LAA has been associated with increased risk for stroke in patients with nonvalvular AF.[32] Some of these anatomic presentations make catheter-based LAA exclusion difficult or impossible. The application of the AtriClip is not limited by these anatomic variations and this represents another indication for total thoracoscopic closure.

It has been reported that the LAA may be causal in up to 30% of AF recurrences after catheter ablation.[33] Because the AtriClip electrically isolates the LAA,[27] total thoracoscopic clip placement may be favorable to endocardial occluders in patients with symptomatic persistent AF to decrease arrhythmia burden.[34]

The advantages of this approach are minimal risk of bleeding, immediate electrical isolation of the LAA, no need for anticoagulation during or after the procedure, and no foreign body in the blood stream.

CONCOMITANT SURGICAL CLOSURE: WHICH CARDIAC SURGICAL PATIENTS SHOULD UNDERGO LEFT ATRIAL APPENDAGE EXCLUSION?

An attempt to examine the advisability of concomitant LAA management in patients with preoperative AF, without preoperative AF, and those without preoperative AF but at high risk of developing postoperative AF is difficult because the literature is not neatly divided into these 3 categories. Also, a variety of LAA surgical management strategies (possessing varying degrees of success) were used. Nevertheless, some conclusions can be drawn from the literature.

Patients with a History of Atrial Fibrillation

In 2009, Dawson and colleagues[35] performed a meta-analysis of 5 studies to determine whether LAA ligation should be performed in cardiac surgery patients with AF. They concluded that, at that time, the evidence was insufficient to support LAA occlusion (LAAO). In contrast, the LAAOS II study examined feasibility of a trial of LAAO during cardiac surgery in patients with AF. The study screened 1880 patients: 10.8% had AF but only 5.2% met eligibility criteria for a study. The investigators concluded that a larger study is feasible, and that larger study is currently underway. In a substudy, the investigators randomized 51 patients to occlusion versus no occlusion. In this small sample there was no difference between the groups in major morbidity or mortality. The investigators concluded that LAA closure is safe.[36] Friedman and colleagues[37] examined 10,524 patients in the STS Adult Cardiac Surgery Database operated on between 2011 and 2012 and for whom they could establish a linkage with the Centers for Medicare & Medicaid Services (CMS) database. The mean age was 76 years, mean CHA_2DS_2-VASc (congestive heart failure; hypertension; age $\geq$75 years; diabetes mellitus; prior stroke, TIA, or thromboembolism; vascular disease; age 65–74 years; sex category) was 4, and 3892 (37%) had LAA closure. After adjustment, LAA closure was associated with lower thromboembolism (stroke/TIA/systemic embolism) (hazard ratio [HR], 0.67), lower all-cause mortality (HR, 0.88), but not lower hemorrhagic stroke rate. In subgroup analysis, this protective effect was seen in patients discharged off OAC but not in those discharged on OAC. In a small series, Johnsrud and colleagues[38] confirmed that, in the presence of OAC, LAA exclusion was not protective against stroke. However, Gupta and colleagues[39] pointed out that this study was far too underpowered to reach any conclusions. An important 2015 meta-analysis of 7 relevant studies examined LAAO in patients with AF who were undergoing a cardiac operation. It included 3653 patients, 1716 of whom underwent LAAO versus 1937 who did not. Stroke incidence was significantly reduced in the LAAO group at 30-day follow-up (0.95% versus 1.9%; odds ratio [OR], 0.46; $P = .005$) and at latest follow-up (1.4% vs 4.1%; OR, 0.48; $P = .01$), compared with the non–LAAO group. Also, the incidence of all-cause mortality was significantly decreased with LAAO (1.9% vs 5%; OR, 0.38; $P = .0003$).[40] This study more than any other was the evidence needed to support a class IIa recommendation that it is reasonable to perform LAA excision or exclusion in conjunction with surgical ablation for AF for longitudinal thromboembolic morbidity prevention.[18]

Taken together, in the presence of baseline AF, the prevailing literature supports LAA exclusion concomitant to another cardiac operation for prophylaxis against stroke and mortality.

Patients Without a History of Atrial Fibrillation

In the Cleveland Clinic study mentioned earlier, 2546 patients underwent LAA exclusion with a variety of techniques for a variety of indications. Five percent (137) underwent TEE for cause at an average of 8 months. After 6 months, there was no significant difference in stroke rate between those who were shown to have successful closure versus those with incomplete closure.[22] In a 2017 Mayo Clinic analysis of 9792 patients undergoing valve or coronary surgery yielded 461 pairs, which were propensity score matched on 28 pretreatment covariates. These patients were analyzed for an association between LAA closure and early postoperative atrial fibrillation (POAF) (AF $\leq$30 days of surgery), ischemic stroke, and mortality. Patients undergoing concomitant ablation were excluded. Fifty-four percent had no history of AF and, unfortunately, there was no subgroup analysis of this group. LAA closure was independently associated with an increased risk of early POAF (adjusted OR, 3.88; 95% confidence interval [CI], 2.89–5.20; $P<.001$). LAA closure did not significantly influence the risk of stroke (adjusted HR, 1.07; 95% CI, 0.72–1.58). LAA closure did not significantly influence mortality (adjusted HR, 0.92; 95% CI, 0.75–1.13).[41]

The most important study to determine whether patients without a history of AF should undergo concomitant LAA exclusion is a 2018 study by Yao and colleagues[42] that evaluated 75,782 coronary or valve patients from January 2009 to April 2017. Of these, 25,721 (33.9%) had preexistent AF and 4374 (5.8%) had LAA exclusion. Mean follow-up was 2.1 years. Overall LAA exclusion was associated with reduced stroke (HR, 0.73; $P = .03$), reduced mortality (HR, 0.71; $P<.001$), higher rates of outpatient visits (HR, 1.70; $P<.001$), higher rate of rehospitalization (HR, 1.13; $P = .002$), and increased risk of postoperative AF (HR, 1.48; $P<.001$). In summary, in patients with preexistent AF, LAAO is associated with decreased mortality, decreased stroke (but not in patients taking OAC), and increased readmissions and outpatient visits. In patients without preexistent AF, LAA exclusion is associated with no reduced mortality, no reduced stroke, increased risk of POAF (HR, 1.46; $P<.001$), and no increase in rates of rehospitalization and outpatient visits.[42] A 2019 meta-analysis of 10 articles including 13,352 patients confirmed that LAA exclusion was associated with lower rates of ischemic stroke and lower all-cause mortality but showed no increase in POAF associated with LAA exclusion.[43]

Taken together, in the absence of baseline AF, the prevailing literature does not support LAA exclusion concomitant with another cardiac operation for prophylaxis against stroke and mortality.

Patients Without a History of Atrial Fibrillation but at Increased Risk for Developing Postoperative Atrial Fibrillation; Future Studies Needed

It has been shown that the $CHADS_2$ (congestive heart failure, hypertension, age, diabetes, prior stroke) and CHA_2DS_2-VASc scores can be used to identify patients at increased risk of POAF.[44] Therefore, a question arises. Can a high-risk group be identified in which concomitant LAA exclusion is efficacious even in the absence of baseline AF? At the current time this seems to be reasonable because the risks are low and the potential benefit is significant. Data are coming soon that should help answer this and other questions. The third Left Atrial Appendage Occlusion During Cardiac Surgery (LAAOS III) study is currently enrolling and will investigate LAA exclusion in cardiac surgical patients with baseline AF and a CHA_2DS_2-VASc score greater than or equal to 2. This study will further define the role of LAA exclusion in patients with baseline AF. The Left Atrial Appendage Exclusion Concomitant to Structural heart Procedures (ATLAS) study examines LAAO in surgical patients without preoperative AF and a CHA_2DS_2-VASc score greater than 2 and a HAS-BLED (hypertension, abnormal renal/liver function, stroke, bleeding history or predisposition, labile International Normalized Ratio, elderly, drugs/alcohol concomitantly) score greater than 3. ATLAS has completed enrollment and data analysis is underway. This trial should help clarify whether LAA exclusion is indicated in patients without baseline AF but at high risk of developing POAF.

SUMMARY

Elimination of the LAA from the systemic circulation is effective prophylaxis against stroke in patients with AF, especially in the absence of OAC. Surgical suture closure methods have an unacceptably high failure rate. In general, surgical exclusion methods recanalize, surgical excision is effective, and the external clip works (when properly applied). Stand-alone surgical LAA exclusion is safe and effective. It is currently underused, but its role is expanding.

Concomitant to another cardiac surgical procedure, there are data to support LAA closure in the presence of preexistent AF. There are no data to support prophylactic closure in the absence of preexistent AF, and it may lead to higher rates of POAF. It seems reasonable to perform LAA exclusion in patient populations without baseline AF but at high risk of POAF. More data are coming to clarify the role of LAA exclusion in patients both without baseline AF and with baseline AF.

DISCLOSURE

Speakers Bureau, AtriCure.

REFERENCES

1. Wolf PA, Abbott RD, Kannel WB. Atrial fibrillation as an independent risk factor for stroke: the Framingham Study. Stroke 1991;22(8):983–8.
2. Chambers BR, Norris JW, Shurvell B, et al. Prognosis of acute stroke. Neurology 1987;37(2):221.
3. Fisher CM. Reducing risks of cerebral embolism. Geriatrics 1979;34(2):59–61.
4. Baker WL, Cios DA, Sander SD, et al. Meta-analysis to assess the quality of warfarin control in atrial fibrillation patients in the United States. J Manag Care Pharm 2009;15(3):244–52.
5. Al-Saady NM, Obel OA, Camm AJ. Left atrial appendage: structure, function, and role in thromboembolism. Heart 1999;82(5):547–54.
6. Blackshear JL, Odell JA. Appendage obliteration to reduce stroke in cardiac surgical patients with atrial fibrillation. Ann Thorac Surg 1996;61(2):755–9.
7. Johnson WD, Ganjoo AK, Stone CD, et al. The left atrial appendage: our most lethal human attachment. Eur J Cardiothorac Surg 2000;17:718–22.
8. Sievert H, Lesh MD, Trepels T, et al. Percutaneous left atrial appendage transcatheter occlusion to prevent stroke in high-risk patients with atrial fibrillation: early clinical experience. Circulation 2002;105(16):1887–91.
9. Holmes DR, Reddy VY, Turi ZG, et al. Percutaneous closure of the left atrial appendage versus warfarin therapy for prevention of stroke in patients with atrial fibrillation: a randomized non-inferiority trial. Lancet 2009;374(9689):534–42.
10. Madden JL. Resection of the left auricular appendix; a prophylaxis for recurrent arterial emboli. J Am Med Assoc 1949;140:769–72.
11. Cox JL, Schuessler RB, Lappas DG, et al. An 81-year clinical experience with surgery for atrial fibrillation. Ann Surg 1996;224(3):267–75.
12. Garcia-Fernandez M, Perez-David E, Quiles J, et al. Role of left atrial appendage obliteration in stroke

reduction in patients with mitral valve prosthesis: a transesophageal echocardiographic study. J Am Coll Cardiol 2003;42:1253–8.

13. Reddy VY, Doshi SK, Sievert H, et al. Percutaneous left atrial appendage closure for stroke prophylaxis in patients with atrial fibrillation: 2.3-year follow-up of the PROTECT AF (Watchman Left Atrial Appendage System for Embolic Protection in Patients with Atrial Fibrillation) trial. Circulation 2013; 127(6):720–9.

14. Holmes DR, Kar S, Price MJ, et al. Prospective randomized evaluation of the Watchman Left Atrial Appendage Closure device in patients with atrial fibrillation versus long-term warfarin therapy: the PREVAIL trial. J Am Coll Cardiol 2014;64(1):1–12.

15. Holmes DR, Lakkireddy DS, Whitlock RP, et al. Left atrial appendage occlusion: opportunities and challenges. J Am Coll Cardiol 2014;63:291–8.

16. Kirchhof P, Benussi S, Kotecha D, et al. 2016 ESC guidelines for the management of atrial fibrillation developed in collaboration with EACTS. Eur Heart J 2016;37:2893–962.

17. January CT, Wann LS, Alpert JS, et al. 2014 AHA/ACC/HRS guideline for the management of patients with atrial fibrillation: executive summary. A Report of the American College of Cardiology/American Heart Association Task Force on Practice Guidelines and the Heart Rhythm Society. Circulation 2014;64: 2246–80.

18. Badhwar V, Rankin JS, Damiano RJ, et al. The Society of Thoracic Surgeons 2017 clinical practice guidelines for the surgical treatment of atrial fibrillation. Ann Thorac Surg 2017;103:329–41.

19. Katz ES, Tsiamtsiouris T, Applebaum RM, et al. Surgical left atrial appendage ligation is frequently incomplete: a transesophageal echocardiographic study. J Am Coll Cardiol 2000; 36(2):468–71.

20. Mohanty S, Di Biase L, Trivedi C, et al. Arrhythmogenicity and thrombogenicity of the residual left following surgical exclusion of the appendage in patients with atrial fibrillation. J Cardiovasc Electrophysiol 2019;30(3):339–47.

21. Healey JS, Crystal E, Lamy A, et al. Left Atrial Appendage Occlusion Study (LAAOS): results of a randomized controlled pilot study of left atrial appendage occlusion during coronary artery bypass surgery in patients at risk for stroke. Am Heart J 2005;50:288–93.

22. Kanderian AS, Gillinov AM, Patterson GB, et al. Success of surgical left atrial appendage closure: assessment by transesophageal echo. J Am Coll Cardiol 2008;52(11):924–9.

23. Aryana A, Singh SM, Singh SK, et al. Surgical suture ligation of the left atrial appendage: outcomes from a single center study. J Innov Card Rhythm Manag 2015;6:2065–72.

24. Romanov A, Pokushalov E, Elesin D, et al. Effect of left atrial appendage excision on procedure outcome in patients with persistent atrial fibrillation undergoing surgical ablation. Heart Rhythm 2016; 13(9):1803–9.

25. Lee R, Kruse J, McGee EC, et al. Late neurologic events after surgery for atrial fibrillation: rare but relevant. Ann Thorac Surg 2013;95:126–32.

26. Schneider B, Stollberger C, Sievers HH. Surgical closure of the left atrial appendage - a beneficial procedure? Cardiology 2005;104:127–32.

27. Starck TA, Mahapatra S, Salzburg SP. Epicardial left atrial clip occlusion also provides the electrical isolation of the left atrial appendage. Interact Cardiovasc Thorac Surg 2012;15(3):416–8.

28. Ailawadi G, Gerdisch MW, Harvey RL. Exclusion of the left atrial appendage with a novel device: early results of a multicenter trial. J Thorac Cardiovasc Surg 2011;142(5):1002–9.

29. Emmert MY, Puippe G, Baumüller S. Safe, effective and durable left atrial appendage clip occlusion in patients with atrial fibrillation undergoing cardiac surgery: first long-term results from a prospective device trial. Eur J Cardiothorac Surg 2014;45(1): 126–31.

30. Calkins H, Hindricks H, Cappato R, et al. 2017 HRS/EHRA/ECAS/APHRS/SOLAECE expert consensus statement on catheter and surgical ablation of atrial fibrillation. Heart Rhythm 2010;14(10):e275–444.

31. Ramlawi B, Bedeir K, Edgerton JR. Totally thoracoscopic closure of the left atrial appendage. Ann Thorac Surg 2019;107:e71–3.

32. Kimura T, Takatsuki S, Inagawa K, et al. Anatomical characteristics of the left atrial appendage in cardiogenic stroke with low $CHADS_2$ scores. Heart Rhythm 2013;10(6):921–5.

33. Di Biase L, Burkhardt JD, Mohanty P, et al. Left atrial appendage: an underrecognized trigger site of atrial fibrillation. Circulation 2010;122(2):109–18.

34. Lakkireddy D, Mahankali AS, Kanmanthareddy A, et al. Left atrial appendage ligation and ablation for persistent atrial fibrillation: the LAALA-AF registry. JACC Clin Electrophysiol 2015;1:153–60.

35. Dawson AG, Asopa S, Dunning J. Should patients undergoing cardiac surgery with atrial fibrillation have left atrial appendage exclusion? Interact Cardiovasc Thorac Surg 2010;10:306–11.

36. Whitlock RP, Vincent J, Blackwell MH, et al. Left atrial appendage occlusion study II (LAAOS II). Can J Cardiol 2013;29:1443–7.

37. Friedman DJ, Piccini JP, Tongong Wang MS, et al. Association between left atrial appendage occlusion and readmission for thromboembolism among patients with atrial fibrillation undergoing concomitant cardiac surgery. JAMA 2018;319(4):365–74.

38. Johnsrud DO, Melduni RM, Lahr B, et al. Evaluation of anticoagulation use and subsequent stroke in

patients with atrial fibrillation after empiric surgical left atrial appendage closure: a retrospective case control study. Clin Cardiol 2018;41(12):1578–82.

39. Gupta S, Belley-Côté EP, Whitlock RP. Underpowered observational studies create confusion regarding clinical impact of surgical interventions. Clin Cardiol 2019;42(4):416.

40. Tsai YC, Phan K, Stine ML, et al. Surgical left atrial appendage occlusion during cardiac surgery for patients with atrial fibrillation: a meta-analysis. Eur J Cardiothorac Surg 2015;47:847–54.

41. Melduni RM, Schaff HV, Lee HC, et al. Impact of left atrial appendage closure during cardiac surgery on the occurrence of early postoperative atrial fibrillation, stroke, and mortality: a propensity score matched analysis of 10,633 patients. Circulation 2017;135:366–78.

42. Yao X, Gersh BJ, Holmes DR, et al. Association of surgical left atrial appendage occlusion with subsequent stroke and mortality among patients undergoing cardiac surgery. JAMA 2018;319(20):2116–26.

43. Ibrahim AM, Tandan N, Koester C, et al. Meta-analysis evaluating outcomes of surgical left atrial appendage occlusion during cardiac surgery. Am J Cardiol 2019;124(8):1218–25.

44. Chua SK, Shyu KG, Lu MJ, et al. Clinical utility of CHADS2 and CHA2DS2-VASc scoring system for predicting postoperative atrial fibrillation after cardiac surgery. J Thorac Cardiovasc Surg 2013; 146(4):919–26.e1.

Left Atrial Appendage Occlusion for Patients with Transcatheter Aortic Valve Replacement, MitraClip, Percutaneous Coronary Intervention, and Ablation for Atrial Fibrillation

Optimizing Long-Term Patient Outcomes

Amar Krishnaswamy, MD[a],*, Oussama Wazni, MD[b], Samir R. Kapadia, MD[c]

KEYWORDS

- Left atrial appendage occlusion • WATCHMAN • Transcatheter aortic valve replacement • MitraClip
- Percutaneous coronary intervention • Atrial fibrillation

KEY POINTS

- Patients with AF undergoing TAVR or MitraClip often present with both high stroke and bleeding risks.
- Patients undergoing complex PCI may require extended duration of dual antiplatelet therapy, which increases the risk of bleeding when combined with antithrombotic therapy for AF.
- Patients undergoing PVI with hope to "cure" AF and stop anticoagulation still present elevated stroke risk due to AF recurrence.
- Each of the above groups of patients may therefore benefit from LAA occlusion.
- Trials are underway to determine whether a staged or combined strategy is preferable for LAAO and other structural cardiac or electrophysiology procedures.

INTRODUCTION

Percutaneous left atrial appendage occlusion (LAAO) is a mature therapy for the prevention of stroke among patients who are poor candidates for long-term anticoagulation.[1] Many patients who seek care for valvular heart disease or coronary artery disease have concomitant atrial fibrillation (AF). Often, these patients demonstrate high risk of both stroke and bleeding. Therefore, a non-anticoagulant method of stroke risk reduction can be an important solution for optimizing their long-term care. In this article, we describe the clinical rationale for LAAO among patients undergoing percutaneous coronary intervention (PCI), transcatheter aortic valve replacement (TAVR), and MitraClip percutaneous mitral valve repair.

---

[a] Interventional Cardiology, Cleveland Clinic, 9500 Euclid Avenue, Desk J2-3, Cleveland, OH 44113, USA;
[b] Cardiac Electrophysiology, Cleveland Clinic, Cleveland, OH, USA; [c] Department of Cardiovascular Medicine, Cleveland Clinic, Cleveland, OH, USA
* Corresponding author.
E-mail address: krishna2@ccf.org

Card Electrophysiol Clin 12 (2020) 117–124
https://doi.org/10.1016/j.ccep.2019.11.006
1877-9182/20/

TRANSCATHETER AORTIC VALVE REPLACEMENT

Aortic valve stenosis is a common valve disease and increases in frequency with age. Over the past decade, TAVR has demonstrated similar or superior outcomes to surgical aortic valve replacement (SAVR) among patients who are anatomically and clinically candidates for both procedures at all levels of the surgical risk spectrum, and superiority to medical therapy for patients who are considered inoperable[2–5] To optimize the care of these patients in the long term, however, we must be cognizant of their stroke risk.

Stroke After Transcatheter Aortic Valve Replacement

Although methods to reduce periprocedural stroke during TAVR is outside the scope of this article, it is important to be aware that there are numerous studies of both pharmacologic therapies and embolic protection devices aimed at reducing this complication. Importantly, although, the rate of stroke in the period between 30 days and 1 year is essentially the same as the periprocedural period and ranges between 2% and 6% in most large trials and commercial registries.[6,7] On average, approximately one-third of patients undergoing TAVR have a history of AF. In addition, although new-onset AF after TAVR is not as common as after SAVR, it is still seen in approximately 15% of patients.[8] Certainly, AF does not represent the only stroke risk factor among this group of generally elderly patients. Most of these patients are over the age of 65 years, have heart failure, and between one-third and one-half have diabetes mellitus, hypertension, and/or vascular disease. Not only are many of these comorbidities themselves independent risk factors for stroke, but they also contribute to a high CHA_2DS_2-VASc score with AF.

Anticoagulant Therapy Among Transcatheter Aortic Valve Replacement Patients

Unfortunately, although these patients would benefit from anticoagulation to abrogate their AF-related stroke risk, the same conditions that result in a high CHADS2-VASc score also contribute to their HAS-BLED score. It is well known that, among patients who have undergone TAVR, major late bleeding (MLB) events carry substantial mortality risk, which is highest for patients with AF to those who have MLB without AF (1-year mortality 48.7% versus 23.9%, respectively; 12.9% for no MLB).[9] Of course, similar to the non-TAVR population, many patients are simply never given anticoagulation due to perceived bleeding risk and most patients may simply demonstrate nonadherence to prescribed anticoagulation.[10] Given the excellent and robust randomized and registry data demonstrating the efficacy of LAAO for patients who are not good candidates for long-term anticoagulation, such as most patients in the current era who undergo TAVR, this is an important therapeutic option.

Rationale for Left Atrial Appendage Occlusion and Clinical Data

Although there is some concern for thrombus located in the left atrial (LA) cavity among patients with valvular heart disease, this stems from the historic data demonstrating LA cavity clot in 30% to 40% of patients with mitral valve stenosis.[11] Our group previously analyzed the transesophageal echocardiograms of patients at Cleveland Clinic with both aortic stenosis (AS) and AF, and found that, in patients who had documented thrombus it was always localized to the LAA.[12] Therefore, LAAO would seem a reasonable strategy for stroke risk reduction in the AS/TAVR population.

Attinger-Toller and colleagues[13] provided procedural and 1-year outcomes in a group of 52 patients who underwent concomitant TAVR and LAAO using the Amplatzer Cardiac Plug (ACP) device compared with 52 patients who underwent isolated TAVR. There were no statistically significant differences in procedural complications, such as stroke, bleeding, acute kidney injury, or death. Although no patients in the TAVR-alone group had a major vascular complication, pericardial tamponade, or (expectedly) ACP embolization, each of these were seen in the combined group (frequency: 3, 1, 1, respectively). More recently, Neitlispach presented data from the TAVR/LAAO trial of 80 patients, 41 of whom underwent combined TAVR and LAAO and 39 of whom underwent TAVR alone.[14] In the per-protocol analysis, there were numerically higher rates of mortality, bleeding, and acute kidney injury among the TAVR-alone group, and a numerically higher rate of stroke in the TAVR/LAAO group (none of these results achieved statistical significance). Superiority of the combined LAAO strategy would not be expected from either of these trials owing to small patient population and limited duration of follow-up.

The WATCH-TAVR trial is currently enrolling with an expected total enrollment of 352 patients randomized in a 1:1 fashion between combined

TAVR and LAAO using the WATCHMAN device and TAVR alone. The primary endpoint is a composite of death, stroke, and bleeding, with important secondary endpoints to include quality of life, procedural costs, rehospitalization, and others. The typical work-flow for the combined procedure is highlighted in **Fig. 1**. At our institution, we perform the TAVR under conscious sedation as usual. Once we have confirmed the optimal valve result, our imaging colleagues introduce the transesophageal echocardiography probe (still under conscious sedation and we exchange the femoral venous sheath used for temporary rapid pacing during TAVR deployment) for the trans-septal puncture (TSP) system. The LAAO procedure is then performed using the standard technique. Once completed, protamine is given to reverse the heparin anticoagulation, all sheaths are removed, and the arterial and venous site Perclose Proglide preclosure sutures are completed. The patient is routinely discharged on the next day.

At the current time, TAVR is primarily performed for patients who are at intermediate or greater surgical risk of SAVR, and who fit the risk profiles for stroke and bleeding that are detailed above. Many of these patients are likely to benefit from LAAO, whether as a combined procedure (not currently reimbursed) or in a staged fashion. As recent studies among low-surgical-risk patients have demonstrated favorable results for TAVR, it may be that those patients have lower rates of AF, lower stroke risk/rates, and better tolerate anticoagulation.[5] Therefore, a strategy of "TAVR plus LAAO" for all patients may be unnecessary, but it is important to keep LAAO in mind as an important option for many of the TAVR patients. Interestingly, there have also been small surgical studies that have demonstrated a benefit to routine appendage closure for patients undergoing elective open-heart surgery irrespective of preoperative AFib status. This may be another data point in the discussion of the potential for benefit with combined TAVR plus LAAO.

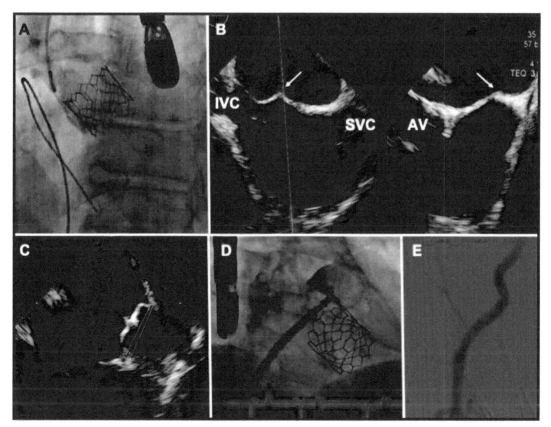

Fig. 1. Typical procedure for combined TAVR and LAAO under conscious sedation. (*A*) TAVR is performed followed by introduction of the transesophageal echocardiography (TEE) probe. (*B*) Biplane TEE demonstrates typical inferior and posterior transseptal puncture. LAAO in position by (*C*) TEE and (*D*) fluoroscopy. (*E*) Removal of TAVR delivery sheath, LAAO delivery sheath, and femoral completion angiography.

MitraClip PERCUTANEOUS MITRAL VALVE REPAIR

Those patients treated with a MitraClip for severe mitral valve regurgitation tend to be elderly and/or have numerous comorbid conditions that contribute to a high CHA_2DS_2-VASc score. Currently, the device is approved by the US Food and Drug Administration (FDA) for the treatment of patients with mitral regurgitation (MR) considered at "extreme risk" for cardiac surgery. Worldwide, more than 60,000 patients have been treated with the MitraClip, and use is expected to increase in the United States given the recent US FDA approval for its use in patients with functional MR.

Stroke Risk After MitraClip

In the commercial ACC/STS transcatheter valve therapy registry, the average age of patients undergoing MitraClip was 83 years, 63% of whom had AF.[15] Similar to the TAVR group of patients who generally have a high CHA_2DS_2-VASc score, many had a previous stroke (9%), hypertension (84%), diabetes (25%), and heart failure (98%). Many of these factors also imply an increased propensity for bleeding through a high HAS-BLED score.

Interestingly, it is possible that the treatment of MR confers a high stroke risk for patients. Nakagami and colleagues[16] analyzed 290 patients with nonrheumatic AF and varying degrees of MR. At 7.4-year follow-up, 68 patients had suffered a stroke. Among the 43 patients with moderate or severe MR, only 4 (10%) had a stroke, whereas 13 of the 52 patients (25%; $P = .047$) with none or mild MR had a stroke. Multivariate analysis demonstrated moderate or more MR as a significantly protective factor (odds ratio = 0.45; 95% CI, 0.20–0.97) for stroke. Although strictly conjectural, it is therefore possible that reducing MR among the high stroke risk group of MitraClip patients could increase their stroke risk.

Rationale for Left Atrial Appendage Occlusion and Clinical Data

There has been concern that the mitral stenosis (MS) resulting from MitraClip placement could abrogate the potential benefit of LAAO in this group of patients. It is important to realize that, among most major series' of MitraClip placement, the average MV gradient after treatment is 4 mm Hg, which does not imply even moderate MS. Furthermore, placement of an LAAO device even with MS (although not an approved indication) may merit consideration in specific clinical scenarios. Among the major studies of MS patients, 47% to 100% of patients demonstrate thrombus confined to the LAA alone (with the rest of patients showing thrombus in the LA cavity or both the LA and the LAA) (**Fig. 2**).[11] Therefore, for those patients who do have MS after MitraClip, occluding the LAA may still provide some benefit with regard to stroke reduction among those for whom anticoagulation is strictly contraindicated.

There are limited data regarding LAAO among this group of patients. Francisco and colleagues[17] described their experience of 5 patients who underwent a combined procedure of WATCHMAN LAAO followed by MitraClip. The TSP was performed in a location to optimize for the clip (high and posterior) and the LAAO was

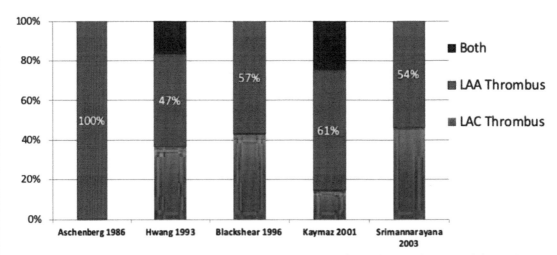

Fig. 2. Location of thrombus in patients with mitral stenosis. LAA, left atrial appendage; LAC, left atrial cavity. (*Data from* Huded C, Krishnaswamy A and Kapadia S. Percutaneous Left Atrial Appendage Closure: is there a Role in Valvular Atrial Fibrillation. J Atr Fibrillation. 2017;9:1524; with permission.)

performed first. The procedure was successful in all patients without any complications and with a good result of both devices. Four of the 5 patients had a mean MV gradient less than 2 mm Hg and one had a gradient of just under 5 mm Hg.

Given the clinical rationale provided above, a trial of combined MitraClip/LAAO is currently in the planning stage. In our practice, we generally advocate performance of the MV repair first to avoid any damage to the LAAO device with manipulation of the MitraClip device. Furthermore, it may be beneficial to confirm the existence of only mild MV gradients before performance of the LAAO, especially in patients who develop moderate or significant MS and could be reasonable candidates for oral anticoagulation.

The prevention of stroke for patients undergoing percutaneous mitral valve treatment is an important therapeutic target. Many of these patients present high stroke and bleeding risk, and LAAO may provide a beneficial alternative to long-term anticoagulation. Future trials are important to confirm the expected safety and efficacy of the combined procedure.

Percutaneous coronary intervention

Approximately 750,000 patients undergo PCI each year.[18] Patients with a coronary stent in place require dual antiplatelet therapy (DAPT) with aspiring (ASA) and a P2Y12 inhibitor (clopidogrel, ticagrelor, or prasugrel) for a duration that may be variable depending on the complexity and extent of the stent procedure, as well as the indication for stenting, and generally ranges from 1 to 12 months. Among patients undergoing PCI, it is estimated that 5% to 10% have AF, many of whom therefore require anticoagulation. However, although oral anticoagulation therapy (OAT) is shown to reduce the risk of stroke or systemic embolization in AF patients, it has not been demonstrated to be effective in reducing stent thrombosis.[19] Many of these patients may, therefore, end up receiving triple antithrombotic therapy (TAT) with DAPT and OAT, which substantially increases bleeding risk.[20] Conversely, Olivier and colleagues[21] demonstrated recently that, among patients with AF undergoing PCI, approximately 50% do not receive OAT in addition to their antiplatelets, despite a relatively high stroke risk with a mean CHA_2DS_2-VASc of 3.6, most likely due to concerns about bleeding risk.

Optimizing Antithrombotic and Antiplatelet Therapy for Percutaneous Coronary Intervention Patients with Atrial Fibrillation

With the knowledge that TAT results in substantially greater bleeding risk, several investigations have been performed to determine whether single antiplatelet therapy alone with OAT is as effective with regard to ischemic endpoints but has improved safety for bleeding. First among these was the WOEST (what is the optimal antiplatelet and anticoagulant therapy in patients with oral anticoagulation and coronary stenting) trial that randomized 573 patients on a vitamin K antagonist (VKA) undergoing PCI to either DAPT with clopidogrel and ASA or clopidogrel alone. Those patients who did not receive ASA demonstrated a 64% relative decrease in bleeding complications. However, the study was not powered for ischemic events so definitive conclusions cannot be made in that regard. Nevertheless, the trial provided the first major evidence for reducing TAT.

In a similar vein, the PIONEER AF-PCI (open-label, randomized, controlled, multicenter study exploring 2 treatment strategies of the direct oral anticoagulant [DOAC] rivaroxaban and a dose-adjusted oral VKA treatment strategy in subjects with AF who undergo PCI) trial randomized patients to one of 3 strategies: low-dose rivaroxaban (15 mg once daily) plus P2Y12 inhibitor, TAT using very low-dose rivaroxaban (2.5 mg twice a day) and DAPT with increase in the dose of rivaroxaban to 15 mg at the time of P2Y12 inhibitor discontinuation, and TAT with VKA plus DAPT. In each of the groups, DAPT duration was prespecified for 1, 6, or 12 months. As expected, the primary endpoint of clinically significant bleeding was reduced by the use of rivaroxaban. However, it should be mentioned that these low doses of rivaroxaban are not approved for stroke prevention in AF and, as in WOEST, the trial lacked the power to identify differences in ischemic endpoints.

Most recently, the AUGUSTUS trial was published and randomized 4614 patients taking P2Y12 inhibitor (93% clopidogrel) in a 2 × 2 strategy to the DOAC apixaban (5 mg twice a day) or VKA and ASA or placebo.[22] This was an important trial to independently assess the safety and efficacy of OAT and antiplatelet therapy, and among the patients 38% were treated with PCI for acute coronary syndrome. Overall, the use of apixaban (compared with VKA) led to a decrease in both bleeding and the combined endpoint of death or hospitalization. As might be expected from the above, the addition of aspirin resulted in a higher rate of bleeding. Both treatment strategies (ie, apixaban and lack of aspirin) resulted in similar ischemic endpoints compared with their comparators, although again the trial was not adequately powered to detect a difference in ischemic outcomes. Taken together, the totality of data seems to imply that, for *most* patients undergoing PCI, a strategy of a single OAT (preferably DOAC) and

P2Y12 inhibitor (usually clopidogrel) is safe and effective in patients with AF who can tolerate long-term anticoagulation.

Patients at High Risk for Stent Thrombosis

As detailed above, many studies have demonstrated the overall safety and efficacy of OAT plus single antiplatelet therapy using a P2Y12 inhibitor, as opposed to TAT, for patients with AF undergoing PCI. However, it is important to appreciate that these studies also have limited enrollment of patients with particularly high risk of stent thrombosis. Especially for these patients who may benefit from prolonged or indefinite DAPT, a non-anticoagulant stroke prevention method (ie, LAAO) may be preferable, outside of the usual indications that include high bleeding risk with OAT alone. These factors are provided in **Box 1**.

Ablation of atrial fibrillation

Stroke prevention after AF ablation is a fundamental aspect of ongoing patient management. The decision to continue or discontinue anticoagulation following an ablation is a complicated one. An important contributing factor is to determine the success or failure of the ablation procedure in preventing future AF. Stopping anticoagulation in a high CHA_2DS_2-VASc patient thought to have no recurrence of AF based on lack of symptoms may put the patient at high risk of stroke. In fact, it is recognized that up to 56% of patients who are perceived to have a successful ablation

actually continue to have asymptomatic AF, thus setting the stage for ill-informed decisions regarding the discontinuation of oral anticoagulation.[23] Therefore, the current HRS/ACC/AHA guidelines recommend oral anticoagulation based on the CHA_2DS_2-VASc score and not on the perceived outcome of ablation.[24] Conversely, continuing anticoagulation in the patient with true nonrecurrence exposes the patient to a needless lifelong strategy of oral anticoagulation and the associated compounded risk of bleeding that increases with age.

Rationale for Left Atrial Appendage Occlusion with or After Pulmonary Vein Isolation

With the above background and given that percutaneous LAAO has been shown to be effective in ischemic stroke prevention and in avoiding bleeding risk, LAAO after AF ablation would seem a reasonable choice. This could address both issues mentioned above: protection from ischemic stroke in high CHA_2DS_2-VASc patients with subclinical AF with a lower bleeding risk and relief from long-term anticoagulation for those who have no AF recurrence. In this regard, a recent meta-analysis suggested that stopping anticoagulation in high CHA_2DS_2-VASc score post-AF ablation patients was associated with a higher stroke risk, and continuation of oral anticoagulation was associated with a higher incidence of intracranial hemorrhage.[23,25,26] Along the same lines, the Society of Thoracic Surgeons provides a class II recommendation for surgical LA appendage closure for patients undergoing a cardiac surgery that includes AF ablation.[27]

From a technical and logistical standpoint, concomitant AF ablation and LAA closure is very attractive given that access to the left atrium is already established. Such a strategy may also decrease resource utilization by compressing all the resources and risks into a single procedure because many of the steps of AF ablation and LAAO are shared. There have been several studies that have explored the feasibility and safety of this approach.[28–30] Phillips and colleagues[31,32] have shown that the combined procedure is associated with excellent short-term and long-term outcomes. In a group of 98 patients with an average CHA_2DS_2-VASc score of 2.6 ± 1.0, the observed stroke risk at 5 years was 0.5% per year among those who underwent AF ablation and LAAO compared with a similar cohort of patients who were not anticoagulated who suffered a stroke rate of 5.1%.[32,33]

The OPTION trial (NCT03795298), which is currently enrolling, will be the largest randomized

---

Box 1
High-risk percutaneous coronary intervention features that may benefit from prolonged dual antiplatelet therapy

Previous stent thrombosis

"Last remaining" coronary

Diffuse multivessel CAD

Chronic kidney disease

Implantation of 3 or more stents

Bifurcation PCI with 2 stents

Total stent length greater than 60 mm

PCI of chronic total occlusion

Abbreviations: CAD, coronary artery disease; PCI, percutaneous coronary intervention.

Adapted from Capodanno et al. Management of Antithrombotic Therapy in Atrial Fibrillation Patients Undergoing PCIJ. J Am Coll Cardiol 2019;74:83-99; with permission.

study to compare continued oral anticoagulation with LAA closure with the next-generation WATCHMAN FLX in 1600 AF ablation patients. It will enroll patients with a CHA_2DS_2-VASc score of 2 or higher in men and 3 or higher in women. LAA occlusion can be concomitant with or within 6 months of previous AF ablation. The primary effectiveness endpoint is a composite of stroke (including ischemic and/or hemorrhagic), all cause death, and systemic embolism at 36 months. The secondary endpoint will test noninferiority for major bleeding. Follow-up is 36 months and the study is planned to conclude in 2021.

In summary combined AF ablation and LAA closure is a logical progression of current AF management to decrease the risk of embolic stroke and bleeding complications on this high-risk population.

SUMMARY

Interventional cardiologists and electrophysiologists perform various procedures to improve the quality and longevity of life for their patients. In this regard, the mitigation of stroke risk in those patients with AF may be ignored when considering the other more acute or urgent situations, such as severe coronary or valvular heart disease requiring treatment or symptomatic AF necessitating ablation. However, we must keep this long-term stroke risk in mind in order to optimize patients' overall outcomes. Percutaneous LAAO may be an important option for those who present with both high stroke and bleeding risk. Currently ongoing studies will help provide objective data in this arena where our subjective assumption of benefit seems well-founded.

REFERENCES

1. Piccini JP, Sievert II, Patel MR. Left atrial appendage occlusion: rationale, evidence, devices, and patient selection. Eur Heart J 2017;38:869–76.
2. Leon MB, Smith CR, Mack M, et al. Transcatheter aortic-valve implantation for aortic stenosis in patients who cannot undergo surgery. N Engl J Med 2010;363:1597–607.
3. Smith CR, Leon MB, Mack MJ, et al. Transcatheter versus surgical aortic-valve replacement in high-risk patients. N Engl J Med 2011;364:2187–98.
4. Leon MB, Smith CR, Mack MJ, et al. Transcatheter or surgical aortic-valve replacement in intermediate-risk patients. N Engl J Med 2016;374:1609–20.
5. Mack MJ, Leon MB, Thourani VH, et al. Transcatheter aortic-valve replacement with a balloon-expandable valve in low-risk patients. N Engl J Med 2019;380:1695–705.
6. Kapadia SR, Huded CP, Kodali SK, et al. Stroke after surgical versus transfemoral transcatheter aortic valve replacement in the PARTNER trial. J Am Coll Cardiol 2018;72:2415–26.
7. Huded CP, Tuzcu EM, Krishnaswamy A, et al. Association between transcatheter aortic valve replacement and early postprocedural stroke. JAMA 2019; 321:2306–15.
8. Kalra R, Patel N, Doshi R, et al. Evaluation of the incidence of new-onset atrial fibrillation after aortic valve replacement. JAMA Intern Med 2019. https://doi.org/10.1001/jamainternmed.2019.0205.
9. Genereux P, Cohen DJ, Mack M, et al. Incidence, predictors, and prognostic impact of late bleeding complications after transcatheter aortic valve replacement. J Am Coll Cardiol 2014;64:2605–15.
10. Manzoor BS, Lee TA, Sharp LK, et al. Real-world adherence and persistence with direct oral anticoagulants in adults with atrial fibrillation. Pharmacotherapy 2017;37:1221–30.
11. Huded C, Krishnaswamy A, Kapadia S. Percutaneous left atrial appendage closure: is there a role in valvular atrial fibrillation. J Atr Fibrillation 2017;9:1524.
12. Parashar A, Sud K, Devgun J, et al. Feasibility of LAA closure for left atrial thrombus in patients with aortic stenosis and AF. J Am Coll Cardiol 2016;68:770–1.
13. Attinger-Toller A, Maisano F, Senn O, et al. "One-Stop Shop": safety of combining transcatheter aortic valve replacement and left atrial appendage occlusion. JACC Cardiovasc Interv 2016;9:1487–95.
14. Neitlispach F. TAVI/LAAO: a randomized trial of left atrial appendage occlusion vs standard medical therapy in patients with atrial fibrillation undergoing transcatheter aortic valve implantation. Transcatheter Valve Therapeutics 2018. Available at: TCTMD.COM. Accessed December 6, 2019.
15. Sorajja P, Mack M, Vemulapalli S, et al. Initial experience with commercial transcatheter mitral valve repair in the United States. J Am Coll Cardiol 2016;67:1129–40.
16. Nakagami H, Yamamoto K, Ikeda U, et al. Mitral regurgitation reduces the risk of stroke in patients with nonrheumatic atrial fibrillation. Am Heart J 1998;136:528–32.
17. Francisco ARG, Infante de Oliveira E, Nobre Menezes M, et al. Combined MitraClip implantation and left atrial appendage occlusion using the Watchman device: a case series from a referral center. Rev Port Cardiol 2017;36:525–32.
18. Acharya T, Salisbury AC, Spertus JA, et al. In-hospital outcomes of percutaneous coronary intervention in America's safety net: insights from the NCDR Cath-PCI Registry. JACC Cardiovasc Interv 2017;10:1475–85.

19. Bertrand ME, Legrand V, Boland J, et al. Randomized multicenter comparison of conventional anticoagulation versus antiplatelet therapy in unplanned and elective coronary stenting. The full anticoagulation versus aspirin and ticlopidine (fantastic) study. Circulation 1998;98:1597–603.

20. Hansen ML, Sorensen R, Clausen MT, et al. Risk of bleeding with single, dual, or triple therapy with warfarin, aspirin, and clopidogrel in patients with atrial fibrillation. Arch Intern Med 2010;170:1433–41.

21. Olivier CB, Fan J, Askari M, et al. Site variation and outcomes for antithrombotic therapy in atrial fibrillation patients after percutaneous coronary intervention. Circ Cardiovasc Interv 2019;12:e007604.

22. Lopes RD, Heizer G, Aronson R, et al. Antithrombotic therapy after acute coronary syndrome or PCI in atrial fibrillation. N Engl J Med 2019;380:1509–24.

23. Verma A, Champagne J, Sapp J, et al. Discerning the incidence of symptomatic and asymptomatic episodes of atrial fibrillation before and after catheter ablation (DISCERN AF): a prospective, multicenter study. JAMA Intern Med 2013;173:149–56.

24. January CT, Wann LS, Calkins H, et al. 2019 AHA/ACC/HRS focused update of the 2014 AHA/ACC/HRS guideline for the management of patients with atrial fibrillation: a report of the American College of Cardiology/American Heart Association Task Force on Clinical Practice Guidelines and the Heart Rhythm Society. Heart Rhythm 2019;16:e66–93.

25. Zhao SX, Ziegler PD, Crawford MH, et al. Evaluation of a clinical score for predicting atrial fibrillation in cryptogenic stroke patients with insertable cardiac monitors: results from the CRYSTAL AF study. Ther Adv Neurol Disord 2019;12. 1756286419842698.

26. Romero J, Cerrud-Rodriguez RC, Diaz JC, et al. Oral anticoagulation after catheter ablation of atrial fibrillation and the associated risk of thromboembolic events and intracranial hemorrhage: a systematic review and meta-analysis. J Cardiovasc Electrophysiol 2019;30:1250–7.

27. Badhwar V, Rankin JS, Damiano RJ Jr, et al. The Society of Thoracic Surgeons 2017 clinical practice guidelines for the surgical treatment of atrial fibrillation. Ann Thorac Surg 2017;103:329–41.

28. Wintgens L, Romanov A, Phillips K, et al. Combined atrial fibrillation ablation and left atrial appendage closure: long-term follow-up from a large multicentre registry. Europace 2018;20:1783–9.

29. Alipour A, Swaans MJ, van Dijk VF, et al. Ablation for atrial fibrillation combined with left atrial appendage closure. JACC Clin Electrophysiol 2015;1:486–95.

30. Calvo N, Salterain N, Arguedas H, et al. Combined catheter ablation and left atrial appendage closure as a hybrid procedure for the treatment of atrial fibrillation. Europace 2015;17:1533–40.

31. Phillips KP, Pokushalov E, Romanov A, et al. Combining Watchman left atrial appendage closure and catheter ablation for atrial fibrillation: multicentre registry results of feasibility and safety during implant and 30 days follow-up. Europace 2018;20:949–55.

32. Phillips KP, Walker DT, Humphries JA. Combined catheter ablation for atrial fibrillation and Watchman(R) left atrial appendage occlusion procedures: five-year experience. J Arrhythm 2016;32:119–26.

33. Jacobs V, May HT, Bair TL, et al. The impact of risk score (CHADS2 versus CHA2DS2-VASc) on long-term outcomes after atrial fibrillation ablation. Heart Rhythm 2015;12:681–6.

What Does the Future Hold?
Ideal Device, Newer Devices, and More

Boris Schmidt, MD*, Stefano Bordignon, MD, Shaojie Chen, MD,
Kyoung Ryul Julian Chun, MD

KEYWORDS

- Left atrial appendage • Occlusion • Device • Stroke

KEY POINTS

- Several procedural steps can be facilitated by using a steerable sheath and by newly designed devices with a closed distal end.
- Optimal sealing results will be achieved by devices with improved conformability or oversized discs.
- The issue of device-related thrombus formation remains unresolved but different coatings of the device surface may mitigate this issue in the future.

INTRODUCTION

Interventional left atrial appendage closure (LAAC) has become an accepted treatment option for atrial fibrillation patients unsuitable for chronic oral anticoagulation.[1] Several randomized studies as well as clinical registries have reported high acute implantation success rates as well as excellent follow-up results in terms of stroke prevention.[2–5]

Nonetheless, several issues remain to be addressed to further improve safety and efficacy of LAAC. This review addresses technical as well as potential engineering aspects of the therapy.

IMPLANTATION PROCEDURE

Most recent registries report acute implantation success rates as high as 98.5% using a single device. Although this may hold true for expert operators, little is known on the number of patients who had already failed LAAC attempts in those registries, on the one hand, and, on the other hand, data may not be extrapolated to less experienced operators. Further facilitation of the implant procedure, therefore, is desirable.

Delivery Sheath

Usually, the sheath used for transseptal puncture has to be exchanged for a device delivery sheath before device deployment. This step of the procedure carries risks for wire dislodgement back into the right atrium necessitating a second transseptal puncture, left atrial perforation (particularly if the guide wire is placed in the left atrial appendage [LAA]), and air embolism. Therefore, it is highly desirable to obviate sheath exchange. Although most of the custom delivery sheathes are preshaped (mostly with 2 angles at 45°) and have a relatively large diameter (12f-14f inner diameter), the LAmbre LAAC device (Lifetech [Shenzhen, China]), comes with a steerable 10F delivery sheath, allowing for transseptal puncture and device deployment without the need for sheath exchange (**Fig. 1**). The length of the transseptal needle has to be adapted to the length of the dilator. In the future, more steerable sheathes for different devices will be available. Prototypes already have been designed exhibiting navigation properties at 2 different sites: a proximal curve that allows for easier navigation to the LAA and a

Cardioangiologisches Centrum Bethanien, AGAPLESION Markus Krankenhaus, Wilhelm-Epstein Strasse 4, Frankfurt/Main 60431, Germany
* Corresponding author.
E-mail address: b.schmidt@ccb.de

Card Electrophysiol Clin 12 (2020) 125–130
https://doi.org/10.1016/j.ccep.2019.11.008
1877-9182/20/© 2019 Elsevier Inc. All rights reserved.

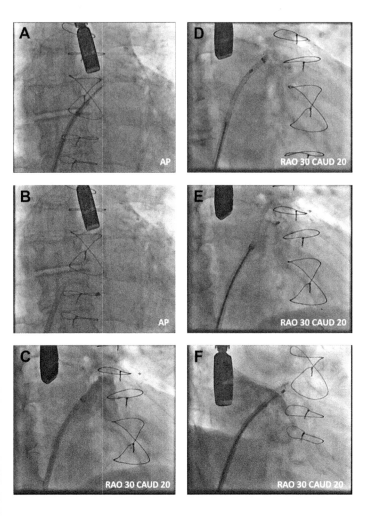

Fig. 1. Transseptal puncture (TSP) and subsequent implantation of a device. (*A*) TSP and (*B*) advancement of the steerable delivery sheath. (*C*) LAA angiography through the sheath and (*D*) navigation to the landing zone with a partially deployed device. (*E*) Deployment and (*F*) final angiography with perfect sealing. AP, anterior-posterior projection; CAUD, caudal angulation; RAO, right anterior oblique.

distal curve to improve device alignment to the LAA axis and minimize torque on the device.

Distal Device Design

Navigation of the delivery sheath to the LAA frequently is performed with a pigtail catheter serving as a protective bumper while advancing the guide catheter. When the pigtail catheter is removed, however, the delivery sheath remains unprotected in the vulnerable LAA, posing a risk for perforation. Both the disc-lobe devices, Amulet (Abbott, Santa Clara, CA) and LAmbre as well as a new-generation plug device, Watchman FLX (Boston Scientific, Boston, MA) offer the option to enter the LAA with a partially deployed ball-shaped device (**Fig. 2**). For this approach, the device is advanced to the tip of the delivery sheath parked in the left superior pulmonary vein. Then the sheath is retracted slowly to allow the distal part of the device forming a ball shape without exposing the anchors. Further retracting the sheath and device

and applying counterclockwise torque, the LAA ostium is engaged more readily. Next, the device can be advanced to the landing zone atraumatically at low risk for perforation. Moreover, given a closed distal end design, the risk for chronic cardiac and/or vascular perforation will likely be reduced.

The implantation technique, described previously, could be helpful in further facilitating the procedure in 2 directions: it has been shown that LAAC can be achieved successfully without a purely fluoroscopy-guided procedure.[6] On the other end, a dominantly echocardiography-guided procedure without the use of contrast media also is feasible (eg, in patients with chronic kidney disease).

Other factors influencing the risk for LAA perforation are the anchor design as well as the device's conformability to the individual anatomy. Although for the Watchman generation 2.5 the rate of pericardial effusion was only 0.7%,[7] a higher incidence was observed in early reports of the

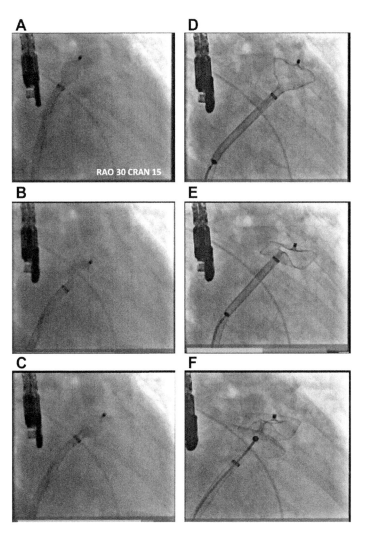

Fig. 2. Closed distal end for atraumatic navigation. Navigation with a partially deployed, ball-shaped device from the (*A*) left superior pulmonary vein to the (*B, C*) LAA. The device lobe is deployed in the (*D, E*) landing zone, and finally the (*F*) disc seals the LAA ostium. Cran, cranial; RAO, right anterior oblique.

WaveCrest (Biosense Webster, Irvine, CA) occluder (personal data). The latter has an active anchor deployment mechanism instead of relying on radial force, such as the devices discussed previously. Another factor for LAA perforation may be a distal open-strut design (eg, Watchman 2.5) resulting in mechanical wall stress to the apical LAA and adjacent structures. Incidental lethal pulmonary artery erosions have been reported.[8] The new-generation Watchman, therefore, was designed with a closed distal end.

Embolization rates for the first-generation Amplatzer Cardiac Plug (Abbott, Santa Clara, CA) were considerable, ranging from 0.8% to 1.9%.[9–11] Therefore, efforts were made to improve device stability by enlarging the depth of the lobe and increasing the number of stabilizing wires. This resulted in substantially lower embolization rates of 0.1% with the current successor device (Amulet).[3]

It seems that the balance between stability and low perforation risk may be optimally achieved with an increased number of anchors at different levels of the device.

POSTIMPLANT CHALLENGES

After successful implantation, the following factors are the major determinants for longer term clinical success: sealing and device-related thrombus (DRT) formation.

Sealing

Subanalyses from early Watchman studies suggested that peridevice leakage less than 5 mm in size is not associated with a higher clinical thromboembolic complication rate.[12] These data, however, rely on transesophageal echocardiographic assessments, and more recent data have shown that cardiac computed tomography is more sensitive for detecting peridevice leaks.[13] Future research is warranted to investigate the impact on clinical events.

Due to the highly variable LAA ostial shape with a majority of LAAs not being perfectly round-shaped, plug devices are prone to an increased rate of peridevice leaks. In turn, large discs covering the LAA ostium may achieve a better sealing. In the absence of reliable comparative data, improved conformability of the plug devices to achieve better device-to-tissue approximation is warranted. In this regard, the new Watchman FLX offers favorable mechanical characteristics that might lead to better outcomes (**Fig. 3**). In addition, the improved compliance of that device may facilitate the sizing process by allowing for broader coverage of landing zone diameters by a single device. Furthermore, some disc-lobe devices offer oversized discs that help seal large orifices on the occasion of cone-shaped LAAs with a small landing zone and a large orifice (**Fig. 4**) or in patients with prominent large lobes requiring coverage.

Device-related Thrombus

Finding the optimal postimplant medication to prevent DRT without increasing bleeding risk is still a search for the holy grail. In Europe, a majority of patients undergo LAAC because of relative or absolute contraindication to long-term oral anticoagulants related to increased bleeding risk. Unfortunately, major bleeding remains the most prevalent complication during follow-up.[14,15] On the other hand, the rates of DRT range from 1.7% to 4% across various reports, and DRT is associated with increased risk for future stroke.[16–19] The specific pathophysiology of DRT remains unknown but seems to relate most commonly to failure of endothelialization of the device or uncovered metal at the attachment site of the device to the delivery catheter. Nowadays, most of the patients are treated with dual antiplatelet therapy for up to 6 months, depending on individual risk. Newer strategies recommend a shorter treatment period (6 weeks),[20] reduction to single antiplatelet therapy,[21] or a low-dose regimen with novel oral anticoagulants.[22] Nonetheless, it would be desirable to be able to avoid antithrombotic medications without increasing the risk for DRT.

With regard to the devices, different coatings could be considered to accelerate surface endothelialization. The Coherex device, for example, is covered by an expanded polytetrafluoroethylene membrane, possibly promoting endothelialization. From in vitro experiments investigating vascular patches, further modification also could be considered, using nanoparticles or heparin/collagen multilayers.[23,24]

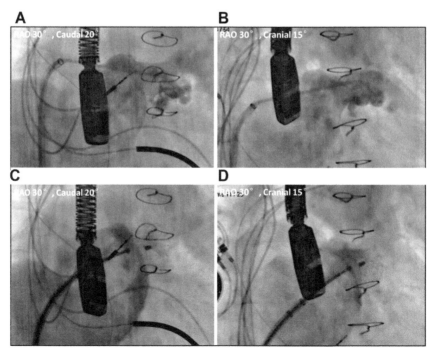

Fig. 3. Small landing zone, large LAA ostium. Implantation of a 26/38-mm device. (A, B) Baseline angiographies show the mismatch between landing zone diameter and the ostial LAA diameter. (C, D) A device with a small umbrella (26 mm) and a large disc (38 m) was deployed to completely cover the LAA. RAO, right anterior oblique.

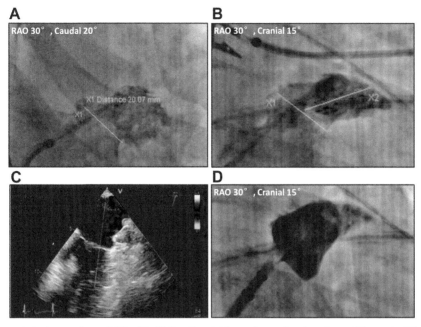

Fig. 4. Increased device conformability. (A, B) Baseline LAA angiography showing a 19 mm to 20 mm landing zone with very proximal trabeculations. (C, D) A 27-mm Watchman FLX is positioned to completely cover the proximal angulations and with a small anterior shoulder. No peridevice flow was observed in transesophageal echocardiography. RAO, right anterior oblique.

SUMMARY

Recent design changes for LAAC devices already have led to a significant improvement by facilitating the procedural workflow (no need for pigtail catheter-guided LAA intubation), moving the workspace from the distal LAA to the landing zone (closed distal end design), and improving device stability (different anchor design). Moreover, the availability of different device types (plug vs disc-lobe design) offers the option to individually tailor the device type to a patient's anatomy; thereby, sealing results have improved substantially.

The issue of DRT has not yet been resolved and deserves future research with the goal of skipping postprocedural antithrombotic medication without increasing the risk for stroke.

DISCLOSURE

B. Schmidt is a consultant to and received speaker honoraria from Boston Scientific, Abbott, and Lifetech. All other authors have no relationship with industry to disclose.

REFERENCES

1. Kirchhof P, Benussi S, Kotecha D, et al. 2016 ESC guidelines for the management of atrial fibrillation developed in collaboration with EACTS. Eur Heart J 2016;37:2893–962.

2. Boersma LVA, Schmidt B, Betts TR, et al. Implant success and safety of left atrial appendage closure with the WATCHMAN device: peri-procedural outcomes from the EWOLUTION registry. Eur Heart J 2016;37:2465–74.

3. Landmesser U, Schmidt B, Nielsen-Kudsk JE, et al. Left atrial appendage occlusion with the AMPLATZER Amulet device: periprocedural and early clinical/echocardiographic data from a global prospective observational study. EuroIntervention 2017;13:867–76.

4. Holmes DR, Reddy VY, Turi ZG, et al. Percutaneous closure of the left atrial appendage versus warfarin therapy for prevention of stroke in patients with atrial fibrillation: a randomised non-inferiority trial. Lancet 2009;374:534–42.

5. Holmes DR, Kar S, Price MJ, et al. Prospective randomized evaluation of the watchman left atrial appendage closure device in patients with atrial fibrillation versus long-term warfarin therapy: the PREVAIL trial. J Am Coll Cardiol 2014;64:1–12.

6. So C-Y, Lam Y-Y, Cheung GS-H, et al. Minimalistic approach to left atrial appendage occlusion using the LAmbre device. JACC Cardiovasc Interv 2018; 11:1113–4.

7. Schmidt B, Betts TR, Sievert H, et al. Incidence of pericardial effusion after left atrial appendage closure: the impact of underlying heart rhythm—Data from the EWOLUTION study. J Cardiovasc Electrophysiol 2018;29:973–8.

8. Sepahpour A, Ng MKC, Storey P, et al. Death from pulmonary artery erosion complicating implantation of percutaneous left atrial appendage occlusion device. Heart Rhythm 2013;10:1810–1.

9. Tzikas A, Shakir S, Gafoor S, et al. Left atrial appendage occlusion for stroke prevention in atrial fibrillation: multicentre experience with the AMPLATZER cardiac plug. EuroIntervention 2016;11:1170–9.

10. Park J-W, Bethencourt A, Sievert H, et al. Left atrial appendage closure with amplatzer cardiac plug in atrial fibrillation: initial european experience. Catheter Cardiovasc Interv 2011;77:700–6.

11. Urena M, Rodés-Cabau J, Freixa X, et al. Percutaneous left atrial appendage closure with the AMPLATZER cardiac plug device in patients with nonvalvular atrial fibrillation and contraindications to anticoagulation therapy. J Am Coll Cardiol 2013; 62:96–102.

12. Viles-Gonzalez JF, Kar S, Douglas P, et al. The clinical impact of incomplete left atrial appendage closure with the Watchman Device in patients with atrial fibrillation: a PROTECT AF (percutaneous closure of the left atrial appendage versus warfarin therapy for prevention of stroke in patients with atrial fibrillation) substudy. J Am Coll Cardiol 2012;59: 923–9.

13. Qamar SR, Jalal S, Nicolaou S, et al. Comparison of cardiac computed tomography angiography and transoesophageal echocardiography for device surveillance after left atrial appendage closure. EuroIntervention 2019;15(8):663–70.

14. Price MJ, Reddy VY, Valderrábano M, et al. Bleeding outcomes after left atrial appendage closure compared with long-term warfarin. JACC Cardiovasc Interv 2015;8:1925–32.

15. Boersma LV, Ince H, Kische S, et al. Evaluating real-world clinical outcomes in atrial fibrillation patients receiving the WATCHMAN left atrial appendage closure technology. Circ Arrhythmia Electrophysiol 2019;12:1–13.

16. Boersma LV, Ince H, Kische S, et al. Efficacy and safety of left atrial appendage closure with WATCHMAN in patients with or without contraindication to oral anticoagulation: 1-year follow-up outcome data of the EWOLUTION trial. Hear Rhythm 2017;14:1302–8.

17. Landmesser U, Tondo C, Camm J, et al. Left atrial appendage occlusion with the AMPLATZER Amulet device: one-year follow-up from the prospective global Amulet observational registry. EuroIntervention 2018;14:e590–7.

18. Dukkipati SR, Kar S, Holmes DR, et al. Device-related thrombus after left atrial appendage closure: incidence, predictors, and outcomes. Circulation 2018;138(9):874–85.

19. Fauchier L, Cinaud A, Brigadeau F, et al. Device-related thrombosis after percutaneous left atrial appendage occlusion for atrial fibrillation. J Am Coll Cardiol 2018;71:1528–36.

20. Weise FK, Bordignon S, Perrotta L, et al. Short-term dual antiplatelet therapy after interventional left atrial appendage closure with different devices. EuroIntervention 2018;13:e2138–46.

21. Korsholm K, Nielsen KM, Jensen JM, et al. Transcatheter left atrial appendage occlusion in patients with atrial fibrillation and a high bleeding risk using aspirin alone for post-implant antithrombotic therapy. EuroIntervention 2017;12:2075–82.

22. Bösche LI, Afshari F, Schöne D, et al. Initial experience with novel oral anticoagulants during the first 45 days after left atrial appendage closure with the watchman device. Clin Cardiol 2015;38:720–4.

23. Zhang J, Wang Y, Liu C, et al. Polyurethane/polyurethane nanoparticle-modified expanded poly(-tetrafluoroethylene) vascular patches promote endothelialization. J Biomed Mater Res A 2018; 106:2131–40.

24. Shan Y, Jia B, Ye M, et al. Application of heparin/collagen-REDV selective active interface on ePTFE films to enhance endothelialization and anticoagulation. Artif Organs 2018;42:824–34.

Moving?